SACRED SEXUALITY

A Manual for Living Bliss

Grail Press

SACRED SEXUALITY
A Manual for Living Bliss

Sacred Sexuality, *A Manual for Living Bliss*

Grail Press

Published by Grail Press • PO Box 2783
Bellingham, WA 98227 • (360) 671-8349

Cover and Interior Design by Robert Lanphear
Illustration by Richard Bulman

Library of Congress Cataloging-in-Publication Data
Mirdad, Michael.
Sacred sexuality: a manual for living bliss / Michael Mirdad.
Library of Congress Control Number: 2005925077
ISBN 0-9740216-0-1
1. Sexuality 2. Tantra 3. Relationships 4. Self-help 5. New Age
I. Title: Sacred Sexuality. II. Title
Third Edition
10 9 8 7 6 5 4 3 2 1

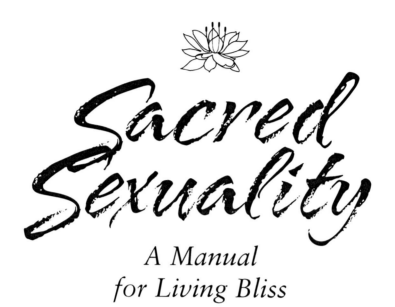

Sacred Sexuality

A Manual
for Living Bliss

MICHAEL MIRDAD

Foreword

Beyond his accomplishments as international spiritual leader, healer, and author, Michael Mirdad is a man with a heart of gold. During our first encounter, the quality that I felt emanating from him was a sense of balance. Michael is confident with a soft humility, serious with a child's playfulness, and complex with a zen-like simplicity. He has the rare ability to take himself and, consequently, his students beyond the titles, categories, and limitations that society or we ourselves tend to erect and into the grace of truth. He is courageously and thoroughly expansive, challenging himself and others to live in the full aliveness of the present moment.

In *Sacred Sexuality*, Michael gently applies such courage to our most vulnerable and intimate of resources: our sexuality. Based on over twenty years as a healer and leader, his approach is simple, yet not easy. It is about walking the balance of saturated ecstasy, while at the same time being nonattached. It is about loving all parts of ourselves and yet knowing that we are so much more than the sum of those parts. Michael's teachings embrace the joy inherent in all aspects of ourselves, our lives, and our worlds. Then they take us even deeper.

Sacred Sexuality eases us through the historical myriads of sexual behaviors, philosophies, and methodologies that span many thousands of years, combining wisdom from both the traditional and the esoteric. By distilling the essence of each, he leads us to an essential truth within ourselves. This truth, which is our birthright, affirms our sexual innocence, forever-expanding aliveness, and giddy bliss. Michael takes us through and beyond technique, teaching us how to apply practical, tangible exercises that allow us to *live* the sacredness of sexuality within our relationships, during our moments alone, and throughout our everyday lives. This book applies equally to those with healthy sexual patterns who seek more profound levels of ecstasy and to those still healing from sexual trauma. From the multi-orgasmic to the non-orgasmic, he considers each man and woman. He honors where we are now and provides the safety for who we know we can become.

Prepare for the profound and ecstatic treats that await your senses in the following pages. *Sacred Sexuality* is not simply a manual for sexuality; it is a manual for living in sexual balance and spiritual grace.

Valerie Brooks,
Author, *Tantric Awakening*

Preface

My personal exploration into sacred sexuality began while I was still in high school. Although I was enjoying sex I found that as I incorporated advanced techniques into my sexual exploration, my early partners seemed overwhelmed, which temporarily left me feeling sexually cautious and apprehensive.

By the late 1970's, I continued studying and exploring whatever information was available on Tantra and other forms of sacred sexuality. Then, after spending several years practicing Taoism and Chinese martial arts, in the early 1980's I incorporated the Taoist concepts of sacred sexuality into my work and practice.

Throughout my marriage (in the 1980's), our sex-life had its "ups and downs," especially since my wife was a survivor of childhood sexual abuse. My experiences with her taught me a great deal about emotional sensitivity and healing, as well as helped me to develop unique techniques related to the healing of sexual issues and traumas and their effects on the body. This knowledge (blended with my experience and training in numerous healing arts) enabled me to integrate sexual healing into my private sessions and my sexuality workshops.

By the 1990's, I was single and reaching another level of sexual maturity. I enjoyed a few intimate friendships and furthered my beliefs and techniques surrounding sacred sexuality. The practice of sacred sexuality (as a teacher and participant) taught me the importance of self-control, personal boundaries, responsibility, and self-empowerment. I have since incorporated these characteristics into my life, my workshops, and this material.

Sacred Sexuality, A Manual for Living Bliss is a culmination of my personal experiences, workshops on sacred sexuality, and more than twenty years of experience as a healer and counselor. Furthermore, this book would not have been possible without my friends, students, and clients, to whom I am eternally grateful.

How This Book is Unique

Sacred Sexuality is a unique book in that it offers insights into how to live ecstatically by awakening your sensual self and sharing this presence with others, moment-by-moment. **This book does not promote *one* particular style of sexuality over another. Instead, it is a synthesis of many of the ancient arts combined with modern principles of sex and sexual healing.** Therefore, you will discover that this book is exciting and enticing, as well as powerful and healing.

Most books on the subject of sexuality are designed to assist couples in enhancing their relationship or lovemaking experience by "spicing things up." They often suggest adding new flavors to the repertoire of a sexual encounter, which, when it works, is usually short-lived. Most books focus on only one type of orgasm–either the physical (masculine–peak) or, more rarely, the soul-level (feminine–valley). This book, however, distinguishes between these two primary types of orgasm and goes on to explain other levels of orgasm that act as bridges between the peak and valley types. This book covers at least *five* levels of orgasm and offers instructions on how to access *all* levels (individually or collectively), thus fully enhancing one's total sexual experience.

The terminology in this material is kept simple to avoid overwhelming the reader with ancient terminology and excessive use of Sanskrit words. One exception to this rule is that throughout most of the book (except the section on anatomy), Sanskrit words are used for the penis (*lingam,* meaning "Wand of Light") and vagina (*yoni,* meaning "Sacred Space").

The genders referred to in this book are typically male and female, but most of the exercises and techniques can be used interchangeably with any gender.

Finally, a challenging and paradoxical point for any book on sacred sexuality involves a focus on the body. While most books on the subject of sacred sexuality emphasize the need for men and women to love and respect their bodies, *this* book maintains that although you must *love* your body, you are *not* your body and, therefore, should not make it your primary focus. You are a *soul*, temporarily using your body as a vehicle of expression on your life's journey. Hence, sacred sexuality is merely a tool for you to re-discover your soul (and the souls of others) by manifesting love *through* your body. Some spiritual teachings insist that you must set aside your body to find your soul. This book, on the other hand, shares the philosophy of *A Course in Miracles*, which suggests that before you can experience *universal* love, you must first remove the obstacles and judgments keeping it veiled. In other words, before you can feel your *universal* body, you must first love every particle of your *physical* body. Then, after lovingly reclaiming your total body and receiving the gift of love from the universe, you will discover that a whole new life awaits you.

Acknowledgements

My prayer of thanksgiving goes out to all of my friends and supporters. Thanks to Lynne Matous for her assistance with editing, as well as Dennis Littleton, N.D. and Joan Koval (Certified Nurse-Midwife) for their expertise. I also want to thank Kelly, Sally, Jackie, Ron, Joelle, Gregg, and everyone else who took the time to assist with editing and proofreading the manuscript. Thanks to the many authors and teachers of sacred sexuality including Valerie Brooks, Mantak Chia, David A. Ramsdale, Osho, and Diana Richardson. I extend my deepest appreciation to all of the students who have attended my sacred sexuality workshops and everyone who added to this book by adding to my life.

I dedicate this book to our Divine Creator and to the Love that permeates all things.

Cover and interior design by
Robert Lanphear

Illustrations by
Richard Bulman
www.BulmanFineArt.com

Table of Contents

Foreword v

Preface vi

How This Book is Unique vii

Acknowledgements ix

PART I • INTRODUCTION

The Sacred Sexual Experience 2

Reclaiming Love, Desire, and Passion 4

The Essentials of Sacred Sexuality 6

The Goals of Sacred Sexuality 7

The *Heights* of Sex Versus the *Depths* of Sex 11

Warning: Sex Feels Good..13

The Complete Orgasmic Experience..15

When Your Body Doesn't Cooperate..18

How to Use This Book 20

PART II • THE HISTORY OF SACRED SEX

The Search for Love 24

Chapter 1 • Ancient Practitioners of Sacred Sexuality

An Overview 27

Tantra 28

Taoist Sexology 34

Sexuality of the Western Mystics 38

Tales of Sacred Sex 40

Chapter 2 • Modern Practices of Sacred Sex

A New Sexual Paradigm..47

Sex Therapy 49

Sexual Healing 50

The Role of a Sexual Partner, Healer or Therapist..............52

The Future of Sacred Sex..54

PART III • SELF-AWARENESS

Getting to Know You 56

Chapter 3 • Your Body

Getting in Touch 61

Personal Hygiene..61
Nutrients and Herbs...62
Hormones 64
Celibacy on the Spiritual Path 65
Masturbation 65
Impotence 66
Anatomy 101 67
Does Size Really Matter?...94
Ejaculation 95
Physical Orgasms 101
Building An Orgasm...102
Exercises for the Body 104

Chapter 4 • Your Energy Systems
Esoteric Anatomy 101..109
Breathing Exercises 113
In-jaculation...117
Energetic Orgasms 119

Chapter 5 • Your Emotions
The Effects of Your First Sexual Experiences................125
Responsibility and Boundaries 126
Dealing With Inhibitions 126
Healing Sexual Trauma 127
Sexual Disorders 128
Emotional Orgasms..129

Chapter 6 • Your Mind
How It All Began 133
My Attitudes About Sex..133
My Self-Image 135
Indulging Fantasies..135
Mental Orgasms...136

Chapter 7 • Your Soul
Being Present..139
Developing Intuitive Skills..140
Accessing the Soul Through the Heart...........................141
Soul-Level (Total-Being) Orgasms 141

Chapter 8 • Your Spirit
Entering the Holy of Holies..147
Spiritual Orgasms...148

PART IV · INTIMACY WITH ANOTHER

Foreplay 152
Initial Contact 153

Chapter 9 · The Environment and Setting the Mood
Getting Things Ready...155
Prayer and Meditation 156
Sensual Accents 156
Awakening the Senses...160

Chapter 10 · Cleansing
The Breath 167
Grooming..167
Cleansing the Body...168

Chapter 11 · Communicating and Connecting
Clarity of Intent 169
Setting the Rules of Engagement 169
Signal Words and Safety Words................................170
Discussing Safe Sex 171
Communicating Your Needs 172
Using Communication to Maintain and Increase Arousal 173
Breathing and Toning: The Two Become One...................175

Chapter 12 · Kissing and Mouthplay
Kissing Breath 177
Biting 177
Licking 168
Primary Types of Mouth Kisses 168

Chapter 13 · Massaging and Caressing
Touching 183
Playful Sexual Exams 184
Scratching and Clawing..184
Sex Toys 185
Lubricants 186
Sensual Massage...188
Energetic Massage..190
Playing the Erogenous Zones 192
Learning to Relax, Receive, and Surrender...............194
Manually Pleasuring Others 195
Manually Pleasuring a Woman..................................200
Manually Pleasuring a Man 211
Pleasuring the Anus (The Shadow Spot) 220

Chapter 14 • Oral Sex
Making Love Using Your Mouth.......................................223
Cunnilingus: Orally Pleasuring a Woman 224
Fellatio: Orally Pleasuring a Man 229

PART V • INTERCOURSE
The Dance of the Divine..238
Choosing a Partner...240

Chapter 15 • Signs of the Times
Reading Your Lover's Response 243

Chapter 16 • Sexual Positions
Five Sets of Positions 247

Chapter 17 • Enhancing Intercourse
Sexploration..255
Variations of Intercourse 257

Chapter 18 • Intercourse for Healing
Sexual Healing Techniques 263
Assisting Orgasms 269
Helping Your Partner Orgasm During Intercourse 271
Causes Behind the Symptoms 272

Chapter 19 • Sacred Sexual Gatherings
The Sacred Puja...275
Sensual Manifestation Ceremony 280

PART VI • THE AFTERGLOW
Postplay 284

Chapter 20 • Closure
Coming Down...285
Remaining Present..285
Holding and Connecting 286
Expressing Gratitude 287
Cleaning Up 287
Communicating..287
Integrating and Grounding..287

PART VII · SUMMARY AND CONCLUSION

Now for the Best Part...292

PART VIII · APPENDIX

An Outline of the Sacred Sexual Experience....................296

Terminology...298

Sexual Facts 302

Sacred Sexuality Workshops..305

Product Information...311

PART I

Introduction

The Sacred Sexual Experience

Imagine how it feels physically, energetically, emotionally, and spiritually to have the love essence of every molecule, atom, and sub-atomic particle in the universe dancing with delight to re-join similar love essences within your being. The energetic response is ecstatic! Practicing sacred sexuality and channeling loving energy are highly effective ways to raise our vibrations to the level of embodied "gods and goddesses."

Science teaches that our physical bodies are not as dense as they appear and that there is more *space* within our bodies than there is *density*. Sacred sexuality is about sharing and exploring an intimate relationship with this inner spaciousness beyond the dense, material body. It's a state of living in the vibration of the soul. It's about accessing our souls–the parts of us that remember bliss beyond measure. Afterwards, everything we do becomes an experience of union with All That Is.

Orgasm is a state where your body is no longer felt as matter; it vibrates like energy, electricity. It vibrates so deeply, from the very foundation, that you completely forget that it is a material thing. In orgasm, you come to this deepest layer of your body where matter no longer exists, just energy waves; you become a dancing energy, vibrating.

–Osho

Technically, all sex is sacred, as are all souls, but not everyone treats it that way. Nevertheless, irresponsible use of sexuality does not remove the sacredness but merely veils our ability to see and experience it. The term *sacred sexuality* has many closely related meanings. But since the word *sacred* refers to "the spirit" and *sexuality* refers to "the body," the two words combined describe a merging of the worlds of spirit and matter, or the soul with the body.

Sacred sexuality is about experiencing levels of ecstatic bliss and unconditional love (usually only attainable through prolonged practice of

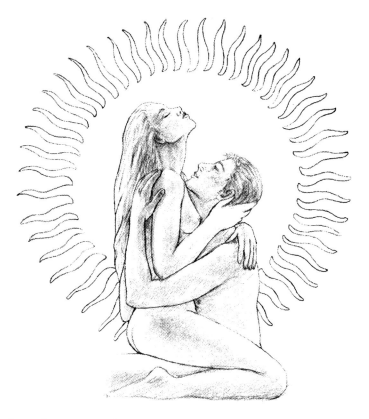

advanced meditation techniques) and, most importantly, bringing these experiences into our daily lives. It's ultimately about *living* bliss and not just *feeling* it. In practicing sacred sexuality, we learn to live *within* the material world while integrating an experience and vibration *beyond* this world–one that feels ecstatic and almost uncontainable. This vibration translates into consistently feeling unconditional love for all people and things, which is why it can be called *living bliss*.

In sacred sexuality, all aspects (physical, energetic, emotional, mental, and spiritual) of our beings are utilized to arouse the fullest sexual experience possible. In other words, these various aspects of consciousness are brought to full awakening and enhanced by the sexual experience: the physical body with its senses and sensations, the energetic body with its energy systems and kundalini, the emotional body with its romance and desires, the mental body with its fantasies and focus, and the spiritual body with its love and divine awareness. All are utilized to increase arousal. Afterwards, each aspect of consciousness, in turn, is brought to another level of awareness.

During a truly sacred sexual experience, our attention moves beyond the sexual anatomy and into the eyes and hearts of our partners. With this higher focus, we become keenly aware that our partners are more than bodies. **As our relationships deepen, it becomes easier to open our hearts and allow our partners into the sacred spaces of our souls.** With the increased depth and sacredness of the sexual experience, passion and spontaneity are not lost. On the contrary, they are enhanced. This deepening trust creates an openness to, and desire for, the experiences of passion and spontaneity. Then, sexual ecstasy occurs at the point when our bodies are merging with spirit, as we disappear as individuals and become one with everything. Contrary to most beliefs, the true practitioners of sacred sexuality are not obsessing on or expecting sexual intercourse. Instead, they are using the act of sensual expression as a means to unveil themselves–on their own or with (one or more) others–and are doing so with the most vulnerable aspect of their beings, their sexual selves.

Anyone who chooses to explore a sacred sexual experience might do so by selecting any part of the repertoire found in this book or by going all the way and applying every one of the steps. Whichever the case, there are a few general stages to any sexual encounter. Although the first few stages are crucial, it is common to neglect the fourth step, postplay (the afterglow), which is as important as any of the others.

In general, there are four potential stages to a sacred sexual experience. Although any single part is enough by itself, the most complete experience goes through the following four stages:

1. Foreplay: building connection and enjoying arousal
2. Intercourse: practicing some form of sexual pleasuring
3. Orgasm: experiencing some level of release
4. Postplay: enjoying the afterglow

Reclaiming Love, Desire, and Passion

Love is both the *goal* of intimacy *and* the ultimate *result* from healthy, intimate sharing. One of the most profound expressions of love is intimacy. *Intimacy* (meaning "in-to-me-see"), therefore, results from the mutual desire to love, the yearning to share, and the willingness to be vulnerable. **Where two or more are gathered with one common goal of love, *there* is the Presence of God.** Sacred sexuality is an ideal meeting place for discovering the greater depths of intimacy. Therefore, how, when, where, and with whom we share sexual expression is worth much consideration.

Since true sexual union is based on harmony, it is important to understand that complete cooperation, communication, and agreement are a must. If the two are truly one, then there will be a great deal of sensitivity for the likes and dislikes of each partner. So, in effect, sexual union can enhance sensitivity and compassion for self and others.

There are three active forces within the human consciousness that assist us in expressing and experiencing profound and intimate relationships with others. These forces are LOVE (with our hearts), DESIRE (with our feelings), and PASSION or sexuality (with our bodies). During intimate relationships with others, most people experience only one or two of these forces at any given time. Yet, the ideal scenario for the deepest experience of soul-sharing between partners is to have all three of these forces in harmonious balance.

Love is what we really are at the level of the soul. To share the heart and soul, we must be evolved enough to hold the presence of love within *our own* hearts, first and foremost. To share heart and soul with another, we must be courageous enough to accept vulnerability at its deepest level, or to love even at the risk of being hurt.

Desire can serve as a bridge between love and sex, or the heart and the body. The desire we feel is an accurate gauge of the vitality and spontaneity present in our lives and relationships. Desire acts as wood for the fire of passion. Desire without love can result in longing and neediness.

Passion and Sexuality are most fully expressed when accompanied by love and healthy desire. *Love* in its healthiest physical manifestation can be referred to as *sacred sexuality*. **In the art of sacred sexuality, the bodies meet to physically express what is felt in the hearts and souls.** This does not mean that all sexual experiences must necessarily be between two individuals who are "in love." Rather, the ideal goal is for both partners to maintain a space of loving presence within *themselves* and responsibly choose with whom to share this love. If both partners *are* emotionally healthy and responsible, this loving presence, in turn, can help to create a sacred union for both to experience.

When we join with others in sexual expression while maintaining a healthy balance of love, desire, and sexual passion, we will experience and share one of life's greatest gifts–an alchemical fusion of spirit and body. But this experience is also contingent upon possessing emotional and spiritual

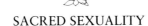

maturity. If maturity is present, we will choose the right partners, those who match our own levels of consciousness.

If you open the door to the magnetic power of friendship,
souls of like vibrations will be attracted to you.

–Paramahansa Yogananda

The Essentials of Sacred Sexuality

A spiritual approach to sexuality can be immensely freeing for anyone who usually focuses on quick orgasms and shallow expressions of sex. Sacred sexuality offers an expansive experience based on mutual love, acceptance, and authenticity.

Sacred sexuality allows us to deepen pleasure, have orgasms in more ways than one, and broaden our ideas of pleasuring beyond, but not excluding, intercourse. It also deepens the purpose of lovemaking beyond bodily connecting to include joining emotionally and spiritually with our partners. **With a willingness to bring our higher selves (hearts and souls) to the sharing of our emotions and bodies, we reach new levels of Divine Presence.**

The practice of sacred sexuality requires the self-awareness and maturity to follow a few simple principles (with love and respect as the foundation) *and* to set healthy boundaries. The essential principles are as follows:

1. *Safety*–You must feel safe and supported at all times. Both partners must be committed to protecting each other's well-being. Safety includes never asking for, or engaging in, any sexual behavior that feels physically or psychologically painful, scary or unsafe. Furthermore, a loving partner would not ask otherwise and will understand if and when you say "NO." Safety also paves the way for open and honest communication.

2. *Responsibility*–You, the practitioner, are in charge of your own beliefs and decisions. In the practice of sacred sexuality, you are the one who decides with whom you share and in what form. So choose well!

3. **Communication**–Once you are healthy enough to create *safety* and mature enough to take *responsibility*, it's time to deepen *communication*. Your needs must be expressed (using words, sounds, and gestures). In sacred sex, communication is done in a loving manner, by showing reverence for the other person and by accentuating the positives. Healthy communication is never judgmental, critical, or condescending, but is loving, sincere, and constructive. Practicing healthy communication encourages you to push through apprehension and express erotic sensations in any form that feels authentic, such as sensual moans and groans.

4. **Trust and Surrender**–Without establishing these few essential principles, or guidelines, you will not feel comfortable enough to completely trust, let go, and surrender. But, within the boundaries of the above guidelines, you will be free to surrender to greater heights and depths of loving, living, and being. Developing greater trust in yourself and your healthy decision-making (as well as your partner's) are major steps on the path to *living bliss*.

The Goals of Sacred Sexuality

If sex, in and of itself, were magical, there would be a lot of enlightened porn-stars in the world. On the contrary, without a spiritual and loving intent, sex limits the expression of our True Self and becomes a form of self-condemnation. In other words, sex without depth of consciousness is not only valueless but destructive as well. Conscious sex, on the other hand, is one of the finest rewards on the path to enlightenment. When practicing sacred, conscious sex, you are encouraged to access the core of love within your being, discover deeper aspects of yourself, and then share with another if you so choose. When sharing sacred sexuality with a partner, you develop a deeper love and respect for each other, while creating and experiencing greater quantities of ecstatic energy throughout the nervous system.

The exploration of sacred sexuality is not a means for self-gratification or the fulfillment of ego-centered goals or pleasures. Instead, it's a method for playfully discovering ways to learn about yourself and others while connecting with Spirit. Paradoxically, this spiritual connection is accomplished by living the Divine *through* your physical life, rather than by *escaping* that same physical life.

When truly walking the "spiritual path," you perceive all things as sacred including sexuality. Perceiving all things as sacred, you no longer evaluate the world and other beings with your senses and then formulate opinions. Instead, you understand and know that all experiences perceived by the physical senses originate in the soul of the perceiver, which frees you to *experience through* your senses, rather than *judging with* them. So every dance you dance (or experience you have) is not really with another person; it simply reflects a meeting with yourself.

If we perceive ourselves as separate from the wholeness of Spirit, we will undoubtedly search for our completion *in* others. This longing to find wholeness through others is an unhealthy manifestation of desire. Once we find the object of our search, for example, we desire to possess it (or them). Now we are approaching the world as predators, seeking to capture anyone or anything that might "complete" us. When one hostage proves unfulfilling, we seek out and capture another person or object. This endless cycle of codependent behavior is the most rampant form of addiction on earth.

Objectifying, or treating other human beings as objects, diminishes them and us. Even Jesus, the Christ, took a moment to explain the limitations of looking upon a woman with objectifying lust. He expressed that **any man who looks at a woman only as a means of fulfillment, does not see the woman herself, but merely an object of potential pleasure. In doing so, he misses the essence of who she is, the treasures she holds in her heart, and the potential their relationship offers.** The same principle applies for how a woman views and treats a man.

Eventually, failing to find fulfillment in others, we begin to realize that what we desire is not an object or person outside of ourselves. What we really desire and long for is a union with God. This realization redefines our old, limiting, negative concepts about desire. It awakens a truer, clearer understanding of the desire to re-member the dis-membered parts of our being.

Finally, we discover that it is futile to excessively displace our desires onto any one person or thing, since desire (as an attribute of love, or God) is a force that exists among all things. Therefore, to single out any one person or thing as the object of our love (when that same love could be felt for all people and things) often makes that very person an obstacle to our experiencing a God-like fluidity of loving consciousness. Nevertheless, we can still choose to demonstrate a unique–even monogamous–love for one person, as this experience can also be a vehicle for developing unconditional love. But even the most amazing monogamous relationship has its potential traps. For example, when a single person (or object) takes an exclusive place in our hearts, we tend to reach for that person with longing, which indicates that we perceive something missing within our own being. In such cases, love is no longer expansive and unconditional, but becomes contracted and fear-based, which always results in pain and suffering.

On the other hand, when our love is directed to *all* beings, *all* life, and *all* space, the flow of our awareness remains expansive. We no longer have a desire to own or control. Instead, we are free to love and be loved–to share love because we *are* love. In this expansive state of being, lack and aloneness are nonexistent. Here, we can make a centered decision to share with one or more people. The ideal is to feel love for all and then choose how, and with whom, to demonstrate this love. To live and love in this state of consciousness is to live and love as God. **Desire is now experienced as a unifying force and vibration felt in and through all things– ultimately experienced as an emotion of God.** Now you are free to observe and relate to a person (or an object) with unconditional, unattached love and acceptance, with no desire for ownership or possession. In such a relationship, there are no agendas, but there *can* be deep sharing. The choice to see clearly, through the eyes of unconditional love, is the choice to see Divinely. Such vision enables the gift of someone's true identity to emerge. Again, accessing this gift involves being with, but not possessing, another person; love is shared between hearts and souls rather than egos.

It is all right to enjoy life; the secret of happiness is not to become attached to anything. Enjoy the smell of the flower, but see God in it.

–Paramahansa Yogananda

This new level of unconditional love and awareness helps you realize that you do not, and cannot, love or hate another because there is no *other* separate from you. Instead, your interactions with others either reflect self-love or self-betrayal. As your understanding of love (of your true goodness) develops, you find that **since everyone you meet is a part of you, you are now safe to love everyone and everything.** As you begin to realize that you *are* love, you no longer participate in needy-love with another. Rather, the love you *are* desires to express and experience itself; and in so doing, this love is expanded. **As you awaken to your natural vibration of love, every particle of universal love is drawn to you.** So as you drink water or breathe air, these activities are no longer perceived as the meeting of your needs. Instead, they are the irresistible joining of two parts of the same whole.

Once you gain a fuller understanding of true, unconditional love, your entire being undergoes a process of awakening. This awakening includes the physical body (sexual anatomy and physiology), energy systems, and emotional body. The awakening of these multiple levels of consciousness is not always chronological or necessarily permanent. Instead, it's much like any other form of evolution: You continually learn, expand, grow, and awaken to newer and deeper levels of awareness.

The practice of sacred sexuality can be summarized as a process designed to deepen your connection to the Spirit of Love and to awaken your physical body–allowing this temple to become as passionate and alive as God originally intended it to be.

The glory of God is human beings fully alive.

–Irenaeus (Bishop of Lyons)

The numerous advantages to developing a healthy sexual life offer incalculable gifts. These advantages include the following:

1. Getting in touch with your own body and soul, which results in...

2. Leading a healthier life with greater self-awareness, which results in...

3. Developing your own healthy boundaries and sexuality, which results in...

4. Awakening deeper connections with the hearts and souls of others, which results in...

5. Developing a greater ability to explore and enjoy the bodies of others, which results in...

6. Reaching deeper levels of love, intimacy, and passion, which results in...

7. Attaining sustained levels of ecstasy and bliss, which results in...

8. Encouraging unconditional love and limitless expansion of consciousness, which results in…

9. Integrating the energy and lessons experienced during all sacred sexual encounters, which results in…

10. Returning to number one and raising each of the aforementioned to a higher level…

The Heights of Sex Versus the Depths of Sex

It's not uncommon for people to describe their more favorable sexual experiences as "great sex." Yet, few have any idea how *great* a sexual experience can be. Those who do, however, would probably find it indescribable because truly great sex involves love, passion, trust, intimacy, and even cosmic experiences. Ironically, according to statistics, what is commonly called "great sex" usually does not occur with established partners or mates, but with someone with whom there is little or no emotional investment. From the standpoint of sacred sexuality, an encounter without *caring* and *feeling* would never be described as a "great" experience.

Even many professional sexologists maintain that the best sex is usually experienced with a temporary lover and not a mate. Unfortunately, for many individuals, this is true. But these misguided individuals have to separate heart from pelvis, spirit from body, and love from sex. Once they get used to this unhealthy behavior, they rarely think to look back to discover what they've missed.

One deceptive aspect of sexual heights is that this type of sexual energy can appear to manifest in people who seem sexually healthy, but their sexual motivation arises from, and is affected by, unhealthy parts of their being. One well-known example is Marilyn Monroe, who projected the image of a sexual goddess but is said to have had a history of sexual abuse that undoubtedly contributed to her claim to have never had an orgasm.

Another example of trouble brewing under the surface of a seemingly healthy sexual nature is that of a woman who is attracted to the "dangerous type" of man. This attraction is not based on "real" love. On the contrary, in an attempt to dance with her demons, the woman feels irresistibly drawn

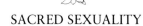

beyond the zone of safety. This very attempt to access and release her repressed emotions is capable of creating sexual stimulation and orgasms. A man and woman assume there is something "special" about an *edgy* relationship because they get so aroused. But some of this *specialness* and orgasmic energy comes from the unseen levels of emotion that are triggered and need to be released.

Generally speaking, **there are two different types of sexual experiences. One focuses on what might be called the "heights of sex," often referred to as "great sex," while the other accesses the "depths" of sex, which is sacred sexuality.** A relationship that emphasizes the *heights* of sex focuses mainly on stimulation and nervous system response. This experience is known as merely "having sex." It is referred to in yogic traditions as *tamas*, or sex of a shallow consciousness. It arises from unfulfilled fantasy and addictive behaviors, rather than from conscious sharing with a partner. It stresses quantity over quality. The heights of the sexual experience are usually measured by the intensity and quantity of stimulation and the success of orgasms, which is like judging the *quality* of food by the *quantity* ingested. Such stimulation has a "hot" energy and is focused on excitation of the clitoris or penis, while the *depths* of sex have a "warm or cool" energy and focus on the ecstasy released between the heart and breasts, as well as the energetic aspects of the genitals. Encounters focusing on the heights of sex could be defined as physically intense and stimulating, but emotionally and spiritually shallow. The heights of sex imply "more is better," which translates as faster and bigger–larger breasts, a bigger penis, harder thrusting, and louder cries of pleasure. These experiences can also be present in the depths of sex, but as a secondary priority and without the need, goal, and obsession for such.

Physical…sex doesn't even come close to the incredible bliss of Heaven…It's very similar to a narcotic. Heaven, on the other hand, is a perfect, indescribable ecstasy that never ceases…Imagine the very peak of a perfect sexual orgasm, except this orgasm never stops. It keeps going on forever with no decrease in its powerful and flawless intensity.

–Gary Renard (*The Disappearance of the Universe*)

A relationship focusing on the *depths* of sex, on the other hand, accesses the soul of both partners. It is known as "making love," and is referred to in yogic traditions as *sattva*, or sex that is wholistic. The depths of sex encourage both partners to make use of their bodies, minds, and souls to access each other's heart. This type of interaction between partners provides the safety to explore the darker issues and inhibitions that may arise during a truly intimate sexual experience. In essence, the depths of sex involve a union of body, mind, and soul. Within this deeper, more authentic sexual experience, heights *can* be attained. Again, all of the great sensations and spontaneity of the heights of sex are possible but from a level of maturity, responsibility, and conscious awareness.

The heights of sex stir us to quickly remove the clothes of our lovers before having sex. The depths of sex encourage us to dress them afterwards. The heights draw us to kiss them numerous times on the way to orgasm, but the depths stir us to kiss them afterwards. The heights stir us to reach for their genitals, but the depths encourage us to reach for their hearts.

Warning: Sex Feels Good

Before proceeding further, it should be noted that both the heights *and* depths of sex can be very addictive. Yet you need not become addicted. On the contrary, the primary purpose of this book is to teach you how to practice spiritual, responsible sex with the goal of using sex to learn about– not escape from–yourself. Sexual addiction and other forms of shallow sex often result from a desire to hide or escape from issues that need healing.

The reason that sexual *depths* can be addictive is easily understandable. Although sexual heights offer intense levels of sexual stimulation that can leave us wanting more, the depths of sex offer a connection of body, mind, and soul that can be all encompassing. In other words, although stimulation can feel good, bliss feels great! Experiencing the depths of sexual bliss, especially for the first time, feels like the voice of God calling us home. There is an undeniable sense of completeness. We long to make this experience an integrated part of our lives. Of course, we can also become attached to anyone (partners, healers or teachers) who assists us in this awakening, but as we make this blissful state a part of our own consciousness, we realize that attaching our feelings to others is pointless.

On the other hand, the potential addictions behind sexual *heights* are rooted in personal dysfunction. **Behind every shallow sexual interaction,** there hides a person who does not want to see or be seen at a deeper level. In such cases, sex is used as a distraction. Despite the obvious physical connection of a sexual encounter, the act itself in this case is used to remain distant from, not join with, another. It makes little difference how intense the attraction might be. In fact, often the stronger the attraction, the stronger the dysfunction. This seeming enigma can be explained by the fact that our egos attract others who appear to have the power to fulfill us or whom we can blame for our lack of happiness and fulfillment. With such a deceptively promising prospect behind relationships, it's no wonder our attractions often manifest as a yearning or ache in the mind, body, and soul.

Hidden behind the potential addiction to sexual depths is a longing to experience heaven. Hidden behind the potential addiction to sexual heights is a decision to remain in hell.

Again, we become distracted by sexual attraction for others as a way to avoid some painful ache within our own beings. Shallow-level sex can be an easy, enticing distraction. The stimulation feels good, but there's a "cat and mouse" ego game involved, whereby we hunt and trap those whom we think will fill our hunger. It's a game for the dysfunctional that takes place in the fantasy of the mind. Although we are guaranteed to go home with someone, we always wake up more alone than the night before. With an intensified level of pain, we try again with someone else, and soon the obsession grows. **Until we realize that *we* are the "other person" we've been looking for, others will eventually leave us feeling empty.**

The shallow or addictive encounter can never produce what it promises. The quality of a building always depends on its blueprint. If you enter an encounter believing you are lacking something, you will experience this very lack. If you bargain away your body to get love, self-worth or anything else, inevitably you will come out empty-handed. It is impossible to discover your True Self (which is Love) by sharing an encounter that lacks love, safety, vulnerability, and emotional honesty. It cannot be done!

Behind every dysfunctional choice, there is a misdirected call for love. It is your cry to the world that you want to find yourself. But you don't know where to look, or you believe that you will not like what you find if you look inside. Nevertheless, be of good cheer. The answer (Love) is as close as your own heart.

The Complete Orgasmic Experience

Every human being is completely unique—physically, energetically, emotionally, mentally, and spiritually. Therefore, the types of orgasms that each human being experiences are unique. In other words, **no two human beings experience exactly the same kinds of orgasm.** Furthermore, no single human being has exactly the same orgasm on more than one occasion.

There are generally two types of orgasm: physical, "peak," and soul-level, "valley." The peak involves *stimulation and excitation* and is goal-oriented. The valley involves *pleasuring and relaxation* and is non-goal-oriented. The peak orgasm involves much effort from the one pleasuring and more tensing and anticipation by the receiver as he or she builds towards orgasm and/or ejaculation. The valley orgasm, on the other hand, involves slower movements and fuller consciousness. There are no distracting goals because the present moment is all that matters. The peak orgasm is quick to reach and quicker to pass. The valley orgasm can take minutes or hours and can last for hours or even days. With a peak, you *have* an orgasm. But with a valley, you *are* orgasmic.

A physical, or peak orgasm is related more to the penis and clitoris, while a full-body, or valley orgasm addresses the whole body including the nerves, organs, blood, glands, and marrow of bones. In a peak orgasm, the energy moves down and out of the body in compliance with the nature to procreate. Most of the sensation and stimulation is around the genitals. On the other hand, with a valley orgasm, the energy moves upward and inward, spreading throughout the body. Furthermore, although valley orgasms have fewer contractions and physical sensations, they take you deeper into your soul. They create a feeling of floating or being filled with liquid or energetic waves. Although external, or peak, orgasms rarely result in internal, or valley, orgasms, it is possible to have both, providing the internal orgasm is given priority.

Both men and women have two separate nerve pathways related to orgasms. These are the pudendal and the pelvic-hypergastric nerve pathways. The pudendal nerve connects to the penis or clitoris, while the pelvic nerve connects to the prostate or G-spot. Additionally, the orgasms originating from these separate nerve pathways are different in that the pudendal (penis and clitoris) orgasm creates a "pulling-up" response in

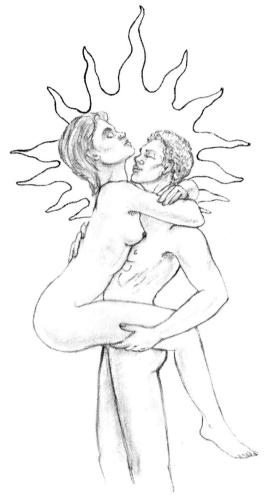

the pelvis (and peak orgasms), while the pelvic-hypergastric (prostate and G-spot) orgasm creates a "pushing down" response (and valley orgasms). Therefore, the level of your orgasms can be consciously affected by the type of stimulation you choose.

There are three other types of orgasm that bridge the seemingly irreconcilable differences between peak and valley orgasms. These bridges are the *energetic* orgasm, the *emotional* orgasm, and the *mental* orgasm. The first stage beyond the physical orgasm is the energetic orgasm–commonly chosen by Taoist practitioners of sacred sexuality. Choosing the level of orgasm you would like to experience involves consciously channeling the sexual energy of the groin upward through the body. Peak or valley orgasms (as well as any other level of orgasm) can be experienced individually or in combination with any other type. Again, you can consciously choose the level, or type, of orgasms you would like to experience or you just allow them to unfold as they may. Whichever the case, all orgasms are wonderful, in part, because they create a sense of openness, vulnerability, release, and connection. Orgasms can also be used to redirect sexual energy into higher levels of consciousness.

SOUL-LEVEL—Depths of Orgasm—Blissful Waves Via the Soul

MENTAL
EMOTIONAL } **—The Bridges of Orgasm—**In-jaculation Via the Mind
ENERGETIC

PHYSICAL—Heights of Orgasm—Ejaculation Via the Body

There is one remaining level of orgasm beyond the description of the first five. This is the SPIRITUAL ORGASM, achieved only through self-discipline and the highest spiritual initiations.

There are seven major levels of initiation in life. Each represents a higher level of consciousness–progressing from the physical to the spiritual. A person's level of initiation can be measured (in part) by the level of orgasm he or she experiences, as each level of orgasm is related to a particular level of consciousness. A physical or energetic orgasm is related to the first level of initiation. An emotional orgasm is related to the second initiation. A mental orgasm is related to the third level of initiation. A soul-level orgasm is related to the fourth initiation (that of the heart). And finally, spiritual orgasms, which are related to the fifth, sixth, and seventh initiations.

7th Initiation
6th Initiation } Spiritual Orgasm
5th Initiation

4th Initiation—Soul-Level Orgasm
3rd Initiation—Mental Orgasm
2nd Initiation—Emotional Orgasm

1st Initiation—Energetic Orgasm
Physical Orgasm

Aside from the various *levels* of orgasm (which correspond to states of human consciousness), there are different *types* of orgasm as well. These include the following:

1. The "not sure if I had one" is a non-distinct sensation that occurs more often for women. This orgasm can include variations of energetic or emotional releases.
2. Peak orgasm (with or without ejaculation).
3. In-jaculations are an evolved form of peak orgasms.
4. Multiple orgasms can be several individual orgasms or many groups of orgasms.
5. Valley orgasms shift from something you *do* (or have done) to something you *experience* as you surrender into blissful waves of ecstasy. They usually manifest as total-being orgasms.

The multiple orgasms mentioned above are usually identified in three of the following forms:

1. Compounded singles: Each orgasm is separated by a partial detumescence.
2. Sequential multiples: Orgasms that are a few minutes apart with little arousal reduction in-between.
3. Consecutive multiples: These are often experienced as one long orgasm separated by only seconds. This type might feel like waves and is sometimes referred to as a plateau because there is no drop in arousal.

When Your Body Doesn't Cooperate

Since most books on sexuality appear to assume that all men and women are orgasmic or even multi-orgasmic, it's important to discuss those individuals whose bodies seem to be shut down. This lack of response might last for a day, or it may be an ongoing issue. If you experience this lack of response, rest assured that you are not alone and that there is hope.

The constant flood of articles and media coverage saying that you are incomplete, not functioning normally, or missing out when you do not experience "sufficient" orgasms is a "double-edged sword." On one hand, it can open your mind to new ideas of what you could add to your life. On the other hand, it can make you feel incomplete as a man or woman and disheartened over the condition of your sexual life. Such feelings are especially prevalent in women.

So let's begin by saying that **every man and woman has had some form of orgasm**. It might have been during sleep. It may have been an unnoticed quiver or perhaps a tear of release forming in the eye. Nevertheless, these responses must be accepted as valid forms of energetic release before greater sensations are experienced.

Comparing your sexual experiences with those of other people is a waste of energy. In fact, a woman is likely to be increasingly frustrated when hearing about women who have multiple orgasms when she can't even manage to have *one* on a consistent basis. It's equally frustrating for a man to hear about other men who manage to make love for prolonged periods without prematurely ejaculating when he cannot make it through the first few minutes. By featuring only success stories, the books and videos on sexuality are very misleading and often leave the reader feeling "left out." But these men and women are not alone. In fact, they are part of a huge majority. After all, only thirty percent of women recently surveyed claimed to have orgasms during intercourse, and only half that number claimed to have ever experienced multiple orgasms. As for men, the average male is said to ejaculate within the first five minutes of intercourse.

There are reasons why some men and women's bodies do not open up to orgasm as easily as others do. These causes include the following:

1. Lack of anatomical knowledge
2. Lack of intuitive sensitivity
3. Lack of patience and relaxation
4. Lack of comfort with a particular partner
5. Unhealed wounds residing in the mind or body

After experiencing repeated frustration from a lack of response to sexual stimulation, a person's body tends to shut down even more. Then the mind and emotions suffer from disappointment, causing a person to lose interest in sex altogether. An often overlooked reason for sexual shutdown in a woman is that women have learned to experience sex like men–thinking that *harder and quicker* is the way to sexual fulfillment. This behavior is contrary to their yin nature, which calls for a deepening, relaxed, fuller experience. In other words, experiencing the heights of sex, with all its flare, passion, and intensity, often has a detrimental affect on a woman's body. It tends to desensitize her, leaving her needing more stimulation the next time. This need progressively increases and becomes a pattern that can eventually lead to sexual shutdown.

There is another common misperception concerning fulfillment that places limitations on orgasm and the sexual experience itself. This misperception is the assumption that ejaculations are the same as orgasms. On the contrary, **an ejaculation is only a physiological manifestation of a deeper experience and is, for many men, the way to escape or avoid the fuller, loving, sacred, orgasmic experience.**

How to Use This Book

It would be difficult to understand and appreciate who you are, your destiny or your True Nature if you omitted any part of yourself, even the most human part–your sexual self. This book takes you on a journey through a vital part of your sacred self–your sexuality. It's similar to a workbook or manual of your sensual anatomy that goes beyond physical anatomy and physiology. It offers explicit, detailed ideas and techniques on how to awaken and integrate your whole being, resulting in a union of your soul with the Spirit of the Divine.

You do not have to be in a relationship to enjoy, apply, and explore sacred sexuality or this book. For this reason, the sections on making love to yourself (which include learning about your own sexuality–inside and out) have been placed before the sections on making love to another.

Even if you are without a partner, you can read and practice nearly every section of this book, especially most of Parts 1-4. This section includes the history and background of sacred sexuality, as well as the topics of self-awareness, awakening the senses, how to create a sensual environment (for self or others), how to pleasure yourself, and how to use your sexual energy to create ecstasy and healing in your body.

The content of this book is divided into several parts. Any single part of this book can be used on its own *or* in combination with any other part *or* all parts can be used. For example, the section on "connection and massage" can be a complete experience in itself or added to the section on "oral pleasuring" or as part of the entire suggested outline. Yet, when combined as one total experience, the possibilities become limitless.

In this book, the term *partner* does not exclusively refer to someone with whom you have a committed relationship. Rather, it refers to the person with whom you are sharing the particular experience. This book includes numerous applicable and effective *exercises* for individuals and *techniques* for partners. The techniques also differ from the exercises in that they are presented in a "step-by-step" sequence.

This book does not encompass all there is to know or learn about sacred sexuality. In fact, the material covers only a fraction of what I know or teach my sexuality workshops. If you wish to expand your knowledge on the subject, I suggest further study of the various ancient arts of sacred sexuality, as well as the more contemporary forms. In the meantime, you will find that this book smoothly progresses from the initial stage of increasing your understanding of sacred sexuality to the fuller experience of practicing sacred sexuality with yourself or others.

Part 1–defines sacred sexuality and explains its goals and criteria.

Part 2–offers historic and modern concepts of sacred sexuality, setting the groundwork and philosophy of this book.

Part 3–educates readers about themselves, which is essential before they can authentically share with another.

Part 4–focuses on how to share the finest forms of intimacy and sexuality with others–from foreplay to oral pleasuring.

Part 5–suggests standard and advanced positions and techniques for intercourse and using sex as a means of healing. It also offers advanced concepts and exercises for those individuals and couples who choose to explore sacred sexuality to a greater extent.

Part 6–focuses on the often-overlooked need to enjoy "postplay" and on learning how to treat "coming down" with sacredness. It also teaches how to make sacred sexuality an integrated part of your life so that the ecstasy of lovemaking accompanies you out of the bedroom and into your daily life.

Part 7-8–offer a summary of the book and an appendix featuring a one-page synopsis of a sacred sexual experience, as well as a glossary of terms and a list of interesting "sexual facts."

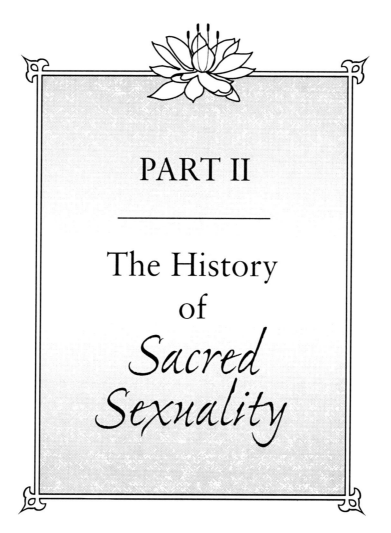

PART II

The History
of
Sacred
Sexuality

The Search for Love

For too many years, we have attempted to deny our bodies and have focused on prayer and meditation as our primary means of self-discovery and communion with the Divine. Now, after suffering the fallout from years of sexual abstinence and repression (expressed in the form of the Dark Ages and Inquisitions), we are beginning to understand that **the completion of the soul's journey is proportionate to our ability to integrate spirituality (the heart) *and* sexuality (the body).**

The acceptance of sacred sexuality has always been a challenge for some, namely the mainstream mind-sets. The various arts of sacred sexuality encourage a personal experience with the Divine, which in turn negates the need for any organized religious system. This sense of liberation that comes to the practitioner of sacred sexuality is one of the reasons every form of fundamental religion (including the extremists within Christianity, Buddhism, Islam, Hinduism, and Judaism) has taught the repression of desire and sensual expression. The most negative blow to spiritual and sexual liberation, however, was dealt to the western world via the dogmas of fundamental Christianity.

The western church conveniently incorporated the story of Adam and Eve as an allegory for sexual temptation causing the "fall from Eden." The apocryphal *Book of Enoch* was then mistranslated to say it was human *females* who sexually tempted "the gods" to fall to the earth from their Heavenly abode. The church used this ancient document to confirm the role of women as sexual "temptresses." St. Augustine (400 A.D.) further convinced the church of the evils of sex. Of course the darker side of our sexual history would not be complete without noting the religious Inquisitions that have left scars on the psyches of human beings even to this day.

Christianity is not exclusively responsible for the veil of darkness that descended over sexuality. Every fundamental philosophy and religion played a part. Yet the root of the problem is deeper still; **the church and state would have no power to restrict our sexual freedom if we ourselves fully embraced it.** Sacred sexuality is our divine birthright. Once we completely accept this aspect of our beings, there will be no institution or thought system that can hold us back.

One of the first dramatic shifts from the sexual dark ages to our modern practice of sacred sexuality resulted from the work of Sigmund Freud. Impacting the scientific community, Freud's work influenced further research into human sexuality and its relevance to psychological health. Although archaic by today's standards, his work was helpful during his time. Another key moment occurred in the late 1940s, when the published findings of Alfred C. Kinsey shattered Freud's ideas of male sexual superiority. Kinsey's research proved that a woman could have orgasms and that they are, at the very least, equal to a man's. He further proved that a woman's clitoris was very much alive and not, as Freud suggested, an atrophied penis.

The next important moment for the evolution of modern sacred sexuality came from the teachings of Wilhelm Reich who wrote *The Function of the Orgasm* (also in the late 1940's). Reich insisted that orgasms are more than just a genital experience. In fact, he went so far as to say that a person's overall health (mind, body, and soul) is proportionate to his or her sexual health. He further stated that **a healthy person could be defined as one who regularly engages in lovingly uninhibited sexual exchanges resulting in a satisfying orgasm.**

Next came the empirically scientific work of Masters and Johnson, whose research, although clinical, helped to make biological sexual response a measurable reality. In contrast to this work was the work of Alexander Lowen, M.D., and John Pierrakos, M.D., co-founders of Bioenergetics, a system of body-centered psychotherapy. Lowen and Pierrakos took Wilhelm Reich's work to a whole new level–that of integration and application–by discovering and teaching exercises to release repressed sexual energy throughout the body.

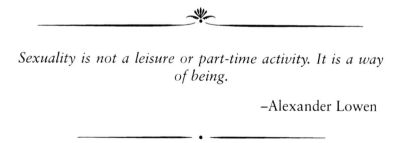

Sexuality is not a leisure or part-time activity. It is a way of being.

–Alexander Lowen

In the early 1980's, researchers Ladas, Whipple, and Perry (co-authors of *The G-spot*) declared the importance of the G-spot and its orgasmic response independent of the clitoris. By the end of the 1980's, Margo

Anand released her groundbreaking book *The Art of Sexual Ecstasy* that offered insights into more fulfilling sexual experiences. This book also boldly revealed the relevance of sexual trauma and the need to release its effects through hands-on sexual healing massage, something that is still taboo for most researchers, healers, and counselors.

After years of sexual confusion and suppression, researchers are substantiating the ancient and modern techniques and beliefs of the practitioners of sacred sexuality. Ironically, most of the wonderful discoveries and insights that modern science has to offer were already known by the ancient practitioners of sacred sexuality.

CHAPTER 1

Ancient Practitioners of Sacred Sex

An Overview

Although humanity has often struggled with sexuality and similarly related issues, there have always been arts and sciences devoted to honoring the sacred, sexual self. In fact, the universe and its origins are steeped in a fusion (or intercourse) of creative forces in cosmic and human forms. All sacred thought systems contain concepts of male and female aspects of this Creative Force. Additionally, every major religion and philosophy has a sect devoted to mysticism. **Each sect of mysticism has a faction devoted to understanding and exploring the deeper concepts behind sacred sexuality and the practical integration of spirituality and sexuality.**

The practice of sacred sexuality dates back to an ancient culture known as the Lemurians. Although there are no known written records of their sexual practices, their methods were kept alive through their descendants, such as the people of the Hawaiian Islands. The Lemurians combined creativity, vibrational healing, aromatherapy, and spirituality. They lived in harmony with body and soul and honored the creative and feminine aspects of life. They were also the originators of the healing art known as Reiki, which was preserved by their descendents in Tibet and surrounding regions. All other ancient arts of sacred sexuality are remnants of those founded by this original race.

The oldest arts of sacred sexuality that *have* been preserved in a relatively complete form are those of Tantra and the Taoist arts of sexology, estimated to be several thousand years old. The western mystics who explored sacred sexuality in the concealed form of alchemy or energetic transmutation came much later. Nevertheless, whatever the name of the sacred art or the time in which it was practiced, the goals have always been the same. The arts of sacred sexuality have always been practiced with the intent of transforming mundane thoughts, feelings, and energy into a higher, spiritualized, personal experience of oneness, or union, with all that exists.

Tantra

Tantra is arguably the oldest known art of sacred sexuality practiced today. The true story of the origins of Tantra is obscure, to say the least. According to legends, Tantra was passed down from spiritual masters who lived in the ancient South Pacific continent of Lemuria that sank beneath the sea, sending survivors to find refuge in Tibet. From this spiritual vortex-like womb, Tantra was introduced to India and re-born in the form of Hindu and Buddhist Tantra—even though the practice of Tantra is usually deemed unacceptable to the fundamentalists of either of these religions (and most other religions for that matter).

Hindu Tantra integrated the practice of yoga, which like Tantra, focuses on liberation and joining. In fact, many of the physically challenging sexual positions of Tantric lovemaking are actually yoga postures (*asanas*) used for personal awakening.

Tantra is similar to the multileveled system of yoga, for both are like a flower with many petals or a gem with many facets. Tantric sex is only one aspect of Tantra. Other facets include the study of sound, visualization, cooking, aromatherapy, and spirituality. One purpose of sexual Tantra is to expand and prolong the physical, energetic, psychological, and spiritual connection between two lovers. Tantric sex brings participants together in such a profound state of oneness and ecstasy that it results in a heightened awareness of the individual practitioner's True Self.

Tantra is a Sanskrit word of two parts. The prefix, *tan*, means "to expand, join or weave." The latter part, *tra*, means "tool." Therefore, the definition of the term *Tantra* has a two-fold meaning—"a tool to expand, liberate, and bring together." The concept of *expansiveness* is one of Tantra's most important precepts. It urges practitioners to push (expand) beyond accepted moral and social limits, judgments, and opinions. In so doing, practitioners demonstrate their beliefs that "There is only God . . . God is only Love and . . . the only rule you should live by is that of sharing love, without limits."

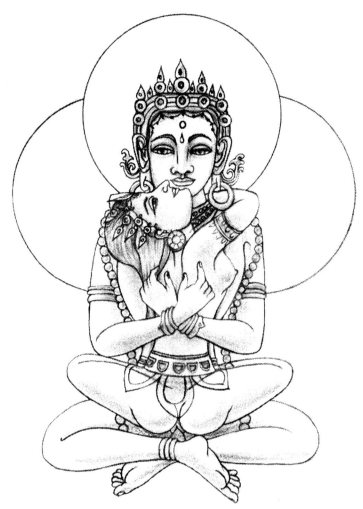

Classic Tantra Deities

Such disregard for the accepted norms of society is what has made Tantra a controversial art since its inception. Tantra reached new levels of controversy by disagreeing with the belief held by most thought systems that we should fear God and earn God's respect through suffering. Instead, Tantra teaches that "Love Divine (or salvation) is not achieved through religious fear and dogma, but through loving, non-judgmental behavior." Practicing Tantra, then, is about expanding beyond limiting, judgmental beliefs.

The most advanced writings on Tantra exist in tantric yoga scriptures and in rare Hindu and Buddhist (particularly Tibetan Buddhist) texts referred to as "Tantras." Nevertheless, the most popular writings describing the practice of Tantra and sacred sexuality are the *Kama Sutra* (Indian, written by Vatsyayana circa the second century A.D.); followed by the *Ananga Ranga* (Indian, written by Kalyanamalla circa 1200 A.D.); and finally, *The Perfumed Garden* (Arabian, written by Sheikh Nefzaoui circa the sixteenth century A.D.). Ultimately, the purest form of Tantra is not passed down in writing, but only through initiations and personal instruction.

How delicious an instrument is woman, when artfully played upon; how capable is she of producing the most exquisite harmony, of executing the most complicated variations of love, and of giving the most divine of erotic pleasures.

–Ananga-Ranga

The *Kama Sutra* was written by a noble man who viewed life as consisting of *dharma* (spiritual substance), *artha* (financial substance), and *kama* (sensual substance). Kama is said to be "the enjoyment of appropriate objects by the five senses . . . assisted by the mind, together with the soul." Thus, the *Kama Sutra* teaches how to attain and maintain sensual pleasure.

Although Tantra might appear to be an art of sexual pleasuring and the *Kama Sutra* a manual of sexual positions, the real goal of kama is to cultivate love and reverence for the person with whom the Tantric experience is shared. Although pleasure is an attribute of practicing Tantra, Tantra represents the attainment of love combined with sensual pleasure. The ancient and wise authors on Tantra viewed sex as something to enjoy playfully, experiment with, and patiently develop. While the ancient *Kama Sutra* teaches sixty-four noble arts that include singing, dancing, drawing, and writing, it also advises studying the 64 aspects of sexual union.

As practiced in the modern Western world, Tantra often is a spin-off of the "free love" of the Sixties–using body movement, breathwork, and various forms of stimulation to achieve higher levels of orgasm or sexuality. Consequently, Tantra is often mistakenly seen as an art geared exclusively toward sexuality. This view is far from accurate. In truth, with genuine Tantra (as with all forms of mysticism) the goal is not about doing or stimulating. Instead, it's about experiencing love without objectification or attachments to a particular person or outcome. Such limitations are seen as constrictions and obstacles to surrendering to Love Absolute.

Although most spiritual disciplines insist that in order to evolve into higher states of consciousness, you must control or deny the senses and lower states of consciousness, Tantra teaches that you cannot experience complete personal and spiritual liberation while restricting any part of your being. Tantra is a profound form of active meditation that expands consciousness using the senses to take you *beyond* the realm of the senses. It always emphasizes the sacredness of sex and sexuality and stresses that there should be no guilt attached to these topics. It teaches that sacred sexuality is a way of deepening intimacy and expanding consciousness, a way to achieve freedom from limitations and to join with the Divine.

Observing a Tantric experience, you might assume you are simply witnessing "great sex." But if you could see the experience clairvoyantly, you would witness an amazing dance of energy and color, not unlike a fireworks display. Furthermore, if you could see into the hearts and souls of the participants, you would observe a consecrated joining of loving intent.

Valerie Brooks, author of *Tantric Awakening*, summarizes the stages of the Tantric lovemaking experience as follows:

1. *Physical: total concentration on the physical pleasure in the moment.*

2. *Emotional: immersion in loving thoughts and worship of your partner's divinity.*

3. *Spiritual: feeling yourself and your partner as a single unit that is connected to Spirit, or God.*

Just as some of the world's greatest spiritual teachers have said that Heaven cannot be accurately described in words, the essence of Tantra cannot be captured in either oral or written words. **To truly understand Tantra, you have to *experience* it.**

In addition to cosmic, mystical experiences, Tantric masters are also interested in having deeply personal interactions with other people and the world in which they live. When a deep interconnection is established, the formerly perceived space between any two people or objects becomes filled with the light of Spirit. This spiritual presence activates and excites the etheric energy within and between the two, joining them as one. That which was contracted and separate is now free to expand and unite. *This* is Tantra!

Genuine Tantra is a spiritual path and is practiced with the reverence reserved for all things sacred. Since Tantra is a spiritual ceremony, as with all forms of worship, there is an acknowledging and honoring of a Divine Being. In Tantra, this deity is reflected and honored in your partner, rather than as an intellectual concept or vague image. Hence, Tantra is not an abstract form of spiritual practice, but a practical one, wherein the experience with the Divine is brought down to the very realm of the senses. Such an experiential process makes it possible to have the tangible, personal relationship with God that is so often sought but not found. Of course, this is not to say that a Tantrika (practitioner of Tanta) cannot choose to practice other forms of spirituality and worship as well, it's just that Tantra challenges lovers to see the Divine Presence of God in and through *each other*.

Since Tantra clearly honors women as manifestations of the divine goddess and sexual energy as a feminine aspect of nature, some practitioners and historians would go so far as to say that Tantra is a goddess religion. Although the goddess, or divine feminine, *is* honored in Tantra and other forms of sacred sexuality, the same is also true for the god, or divine masculine. To accentuate only the goddess promotes imbalance in the universe. A deeper understanding of the principles of polarity reveals that ideally *both* genders should be equally honored. When honored completely and unconditionally, they eventual merge into *one* where there is no longer a distinction between male and female.

Although Tantra incorporates ceremony and ritual and involves the worshiping or honoring of a Divine Creative Source (as the Divine aspect found within all beings), it is not like any *formal* religion. It has no hierarchy or rigidity within its rituals and is centered in the heart rather than dogma. Its roots, or origins, can no more be claimed by Hindu or Buddhist than the origins of Sufism can be claimed by Islam; Christ Consciousness, by the fundamental Christian; or Kabbalah, by the Jew.

Tantra has two distinct paths of training, a left-hand path (*vama-marga*) and a right-hand path (*dakshina-marga*). The left-hand path practices a more literal form of Tantra that usually involves intercourse, while the right-hand path practices a symbolic form of Tantra that views intercourse as an allegory. The left-hand path of Tantra practices the *maithuna* ritual known as "The Five *Makaras*." During an evening gathering, several practitioners join to partake of the five symbols of pleasure, which are *madya* (wine), *matsya* (fish), *mamsa* (meat), *mudra* (parched grain), and *maithuna* (sacred sex). Practitioners of left-hand path Tantra also vary from one group to another in that some focus more on spirituality, others on energy (even magic), others on sensuality, and still others on a blend of the above.

In Tantric writings, a woman's sexual and spiritual energies are often referred to as "shakti." In Hindu traditions the goddess Shakti represents the female principle or energy. Although the female force, or shakti, exists in both women and men, women are seen as the "guardians" of the shakti energy. According to ancient Tantric writings, the power of the shakti is limitless. Once awakened, this spiritual, energetic, and sexual force can be channeled creatively.

Upon awakening, Shakti rises up the spine to meet Shiva, her male counterpart. Together their merged energies create an alchemical fusion of bliss. Thus in Tantra, the coupling of a man and woman serves to represent the greater, universal creative process, as the intercourse between a couple simulates the creation dance of Shakti and Shiva.

Ironically, irrespective of its depth and purpose, *Tantra* has become such a common term that it is used to market everything from sex and videos to jewelry and sensual oils. Despite misrepresentations to the contrary, Tantra is a system of spiritual mysticism *and* personal experience, not exclusively a sexual art.

The primary components for practicing *authentic* Tantra include various forms of meditation and kundalini yoga. More specifically, Tantra incorporates *asanas* (yoga postures), *pranayama* (specific breathing techniques), *mantras* (repetition of sacred syllables), *yantras* (visualization), and *bandhas* (muscular energy locks). Tantric breathing and mind focusing exercises are very effective in adding to *any* truly sacred experience. Yet, as with all things, it is possible to become too caught up in the techniques, whereby they become distractions, rather than valuable tools.

Tantric masters see no fundamental difference between themselves and their students. Since both are equally valuable, the ideal arrangement is to create the most intimate possible relationship between master and student, but without the worship of, or obsession on, the person. This viewpoint encourages relationships that are loving, alive, playful, and honest. In fact, Tantric masters see their students as so valuable that they often limit their number to a minimum, assuring a greater quality of personal and individual contact. These relationships are so personal that in India the students often live with or nearby their masters' families. Rather than having ashrams and temples, the masters use their own homes, preferring a more intimate environment.

Tantra is not to be confused with other arts of sacred sexuality, including Taoist sexual practices. Although different, Tantra (from India) and Taoism (from China) share some similar concepts. Both involve balancing the male

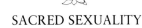

and female energies. What Tantra calls the dance of Shakti and Shiva, Taoists call the balancing of yin and yang. Both systems have a goal of total physical and spiritual union, for Tantra and Taoism are each an ancient form of sacred sexuality. In both traditions, sexuality is practiced in a spiritual context.

Nevertheless, the differences are very distinct. For example, Tantra uses more ceremony and ritual, while Taoism is more scientific or methodical and focuses on the body, its meridians, and energy systems. Tantra emphasizes the *art* of sex, while Taoist sexology emphasizes the *science*. In Tantra there is less emphasis on "controlling orgasms" by "constricting specific muscles." Instead, in the art of Tantra there is emphasis on relaxing into the orgasmic sensations, rather than tensing in any form. On the other hand, in the Taoist sexual systems, control and muscle constriction are at the very heart of the techniques and principles. Although Tantrikas may not agree with all Taoist concepts of ejaculation control, Taoists have developed their principles of sexuality into a science that has worked for thousands of years. Taoist masters, who are commonly known to live in vibrant health for well over a hundred years, attribute their semi-immortality to their sexual practices of ejaculation control and in-jaculation.

Because of the differences between Tantric and Taoist sexual practices, most practitioners of any ancient system of sexuality follow only *one* of these two paths. Few practitioners have learned to reconcile, synthesize, and integrate the two. Nevertheless, the key to successfully practicing sacred sexuality is to use *both* techniques at precisely the right moment.

Taoist Sexology

Although Taoism (pronounced Dow-ism), as a philosophy or religion in China, developed later than the Hindu religion of India, both traditions embraced some form of sacred sexuality. The Chinese sexual arts were developed by the Yellow Emperor (Huang-Ti) and his "three immortal ladies" long before Taoism, which means that although Hinduism is older than Taoism, the Chinese sexual arts are still as ancient as Tantra.

Like Tantra, Taoism has many facets, sex being only one of eight "spokes to their wheel." Royalty often consulted the wise and respected Taoist masters on issues related to philosophy, health, life, and sex. Some of these teachings were preserved and are known as "Canons of Wisdom." The most common set of ancient writings on Taoist lovemaking is called the "pillow books."

The various eight facets of Taoism are known as the "Eight Disciplines" and are as follows:

1. **Tao of Philosophy**–focuses on the metaphysics of life and suggestions for spiritual elevation.

2. **Tao of Sexual Wisdom**–teaches the use of sexual exercises and sexual energy to improve health and vitality.

3. **Tao of Balanced Diet**–relates to diet, food preparation, and the importance of keeping an acid/alkaline balance.

4. **Tao of Mastery**–develops use of such ancient divination tools as face reading, astrology, numerology, and symbology.

5. **Tao of Success**–features the study of natural forces through the mathematical sciences of geometry and physics, as well as the use of the I Ching.

6. **Tao of Revitalization**–offers a routine of internal exercises directing healing power into the body.

7. **Tao of Healing Art**–includes the art of healing others through massage and various hands-on healing arts.

8. **Tao of Forgotten Food Diet**–educates in the use of herbs for healing and as supplements.

The primary purpose behind Taoist lovemaking is the transformation of sexual energy into healing energy and vitality, resulting in better health and potential immortality. The primary Taoist technique to achieve these healing effects is called the inward orgasm (in-jaculation), whereby the orgasmic energy rises up the spine, stimulating the endocrine glands, energy systems, nervous system, and organs. **Taoists teach that an inner orgasm (in-jaculation) stimulates life and vitality, while the outer orgasm (e-jaculation) brings death or loss of health and vitality.** An in-jaculation is the most effective tool for transforming a physical orgasm into an energetic orgasm. Of course, there are even higher levels of orgasm as well, including a soul-level, total-being orgasm.

Taoist self-transformation exercises are designed to bring the practitioner to a state of immortality by cultivating what they refer to as the three energies, or "Three Treasures." The first is *ching* (sexual and physical energy), the second is *qi* (etheric and breath energy), and the third is *shen* (mental and spiritual energy). Only with sufficient *ching* can the body produce sufficient *qi*. Then, with sufficient *qi*, a balance of *shen* is restored. These three essences must be restored and refined to their optimum level

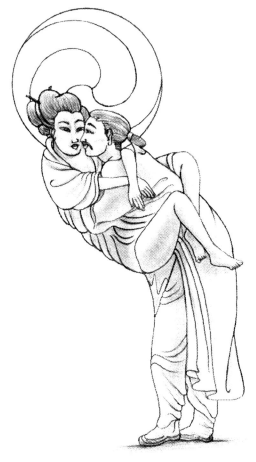

Classic Taoist lovers

and balance to attain the gifts of the "Three Treasures," or the "Elixir of Immortality." Practitioners of Taoist sexuality believe that sexual energy is the most powerful human energy and that the use of sexual rejuvenation and in-jaculation techniques are the most effective and efficient way to revitalize and develop these "Three Treasures."

Taoists gauge a person's vital life-force by the "measures" of positive energy that he or she possesses. These measures can be increased or decreased. The Taoist master Chao Pi Ch'en taught that if a person consciously and consistently develops his life-force for one hundred days, he will gain sixty-four measures of chi. If he continues another one hundred successive days, the practitioner will feel healthier, and aliments will disappear. If he practices for another one hundred days, he will feel vibrant and light. Finally, if he continues, his hair will be restored, and lost teeth will grow back.

Taoists use imaginative, and sometimes humorous, metaphors to illustrate their concepts about sexuality. For example, they regard man as fire and woman as water. Fire, once started, burns fast and can burn out, when, on the other hand, the woman (or water) is just beginning to boil (or get hot). Therefore, the man must control his fire to prolong his climax (and erection). Then he can help the woman reach her natural stages of warming up toward orgasm, thus enhancing the experience for both partners.

Again, Taoists say that the male is like fire and the woman is like water. The man's fire (penis or lingam) boils the woman's water (her womb or yoni). If the man is *not* trained in the art of lovemaking, her water will extinguish his fire. Thus, the soft and yielding (yin) can conquer the hard (yang), just as the proverbial flowing river conquers the hardest of rocks.

Taoists do not merely teach exercises to enhance the pleasure of partnership. They also encourage self-mastery and self-awareness for improved health and vitality. They clearly teach the importance of drawing in the sexual energy and experience, rather than focusing on sexual organs and external stimuli. Any focus on the sexual organs is used only to introduce the practitioner to more advanced concepts. Taoist master Mantak Chia says that the goal of Taoist sexual practices is like that of making chicken broth: If you boil a chicken in water and extract the vital essence into the water, which is more valuable, the chicken or the broth? Clearly, **the Taoists believe the valuable energy generated during lovemaking is more vital to one's well-being than the stimulation to the organs.**

In the Taoist tradition, sexual energy is nurtured and valued for its role in the overall well-being of the body, mind, and spirit. It is the water of life, or life-giving essence, for all that exists in the material world. Taoists see sexual energy as the fuel behind the body's chi (energy, vital essence or life-force). Stimulation of the sexual organs and sex glands enhances this life-force and thereby encourages the secretion of hormones from the other major endocrine glands (adrenal, thymus, thyroid, pituitary, and pineal). Therefore, Taoist sexual exercises assist in the production of potent hormones and stimulate the healthy function of the endocrine glands, the master controls of the body.

The legendary Yellow Emperor recorded conversations with Taoist advisors on many subjects. Their works include *Classic of the Plain Girl* (Arcane Maid) and *Counsels of a Simple Girl*. Within these writings, the Taoist sages use metaphors of combat to describe the act of sex, which is fitting because sex engages so many energies and physical movements.

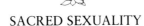

Thus, Taoists warn the male not to be too aggressive by ambitiously attacking and throwing away his spear (discharging his sperm), like a warrior wasting ammunition. Otherwise, he will find himself unarmed and will have to run away.

Another metaphor of battle says that a woman has a shield (vaginal lips) and a short sword (clitoris). So, to truly engage with his opponent (partner), a man must use short-range weapons (fingers, hands, and tongue). His long-range weapon (penis) should be used to entice his partner and then brought out only after he has weakened her, and she is prepared to surrender. Finally, she yields because he has won her trust and respect by his demonstration of self-control. Now they are ready for an equal, intimate level of engagement.

Taoists treat sex as a healing art. Since the hands are considered primary channels of energy, they are used in various positions and techniques to assist in lovemaking. For example, during a sexual encounter, the hands (charged with healing energy) are placed over areas that lack vitality or seem to need healing.

Another example of blending the use of healing with sexuality involves recognizing that the partner doing the moving is bringing healing to the partner who is lying (or sitting) still. Since Taoists encourage the awareness and use of healing energy for both partners, **alternating active roles during a sexual encounter is necessarily vital to achieving equal opportunities for healing.**

According to Taoist philosophy, the male often burns himself out from taking the more active, assertive sexual role and/or reaching climax too quickly. Taoist masters, therefore, instruct the woman to share the physical exerting and the man to occasionally cease all forms of stimulation to his penis to avoid becoming overly aroused. Instead, he is to delay his orgasm, even to the point of occasionally avoiding ejaculation altogether.

Taoists are emphatic about the value of semen retention, or in-jaculation. The ancient Taoist masters referred to a ten-day process that procured the invaluable results of ejaculation retention. In one ancient text they wrote:

"If a man has intercourse once without spilling his seed, his vital essence is strengthened. If he does this twice, his vision and hearing are made clearer. If three times, his physical illnesses will begin to disappear. The fourth time he will begin to feel inner peace. The fifth time his blood will circulate powerfully. The sixth time his genitals will gain new prowess. By

the seventh his thighs and buttock (muscles and meridians) will become firm. The eighth time his entire body will radiate good health. The ninth time his life-span will be increased." –Canon of Taoist Wisdom

Sexuality of the Western Mystics

Since the human etheric body is very similar to that of plants, the ancient Native Americans had a ritual for revitalization of the human energy field by hugging a tree. The same principle of rejuvenation applies to a child who instinctively rolls around in the grass. Like the Native Americans, the ancient Essenes (an ascetic group of mystics that lived in the Judean region long before, and up until, the time of Christ) also had a ritual whereby they revitalized themselves. They used exercises that would transform their sexual energy into a usable force for growth and well-being. During these rituals they prayed, "Angel of Life, enter my generative organs and regenerate my whole body."

According to some of the Essene manuscripts, **the masters in the Essene community were more apt to achieve transmutation of energy by thought, while the students still used the more physical rituals for stimulation, arousal, and transmutation.** For example, the students would stimulate sex organs with a "mini-generator" made of wheat grass.

Edmond Bordeaux, translator of *The Essene Gospel of Peace* and father of modern Essene studies, used this *biogenic* sexual-rejuvenation grass technique at his ranch in Costa Rica. A man massaged his penis with fresh sprouts, while a woman used the sprouts to massage her breasts, vagina, and clitoris to achieve stimulation. Nearly ninety percent of the participants reported a noticeable change in their overall vitality. Their testimonies also noted an enhancement in their orgasms when using their portable organic "battery" in foreplay.

Long after the disappearance of the mystic-Essenes, the art of sacred sexuality (during the Middle Ages) was known as *alchemy*, meaning "All-Chemistry" or "God's Chemistry." This lost science was said to have been the art of transmuting base metals into gold.

It's now understood that the western mystics were actually using metaphor to discuss their art of sacred sexuality. They were describing the transmutation of base, sexual energy into valuable, ecstatic, soul-level orgasms.

Common tools of the alchemist include the pestle and mortar, which are symbols of a lingam and yoni. Here, the grinding activity between the two represents sexual union. Other tools of the alchemist are the wand and cistern or knife and bowl. Again these symbolize the creative activity between the male and female principles, or the lingam and yoni. Furthermore, these **symbols of sexual union represent the creative mind piercing and activating the receptive void, just as the Spirit of God moved upon the face of the deep.**

Unfortunately, some practitioners of what is commonly referred to as sex magic or alchemical sex have a different focus. Their goal is ego self-gratification, not joining in oneness. While all practitioners of sex magic may not be ego-centered, many of them *are* known to maintain a detachment from their lovers and use them as mere tools to ignite their own energetic systems. Lacking true intimacy and spiritual depth, however, their sexual encounters can never be confused with anything sacred–particularly sacred sexuality.

Tales of Sacred Sex

The following are myths, legends, and stories of sacred sexuality from numerous cultures throughout history. Each legend possesses valuable insights into the meaning of sacred sexuality.

ACTAEON AND DIANA

When Actaeon, (a respected hunter who symbolizes the physical self) happened upon the great goddess Diana, naked and washing herself, he failed to fall down and worship her. Instead, he chose to make a sexual advance. Because he failed to see and honor her divinity, she turned him into a stag (symbolizing his out-of-control horniness). Afterwards, Actaeon's own hunting dogs devoured him. This story suggests that when our sexual desires are out of control and we fail to recognize the sacred spirit within that which we desire, our actions will inevitably destroy us.

CUPID AND PSYCHE

The story of Cupid and Psyche offers deep insights into the connection between eroticism and spirituality. Cupid, who is also known as Eros, or Amour, is the god of erotic love, and Psyche represents the beauty of the soul.

When the goddess Venus becomes jealous of Psyche's beauty, Venus asks Eros to cause Psyche to fall in love with some unworthy man. Instead, Eros takes Psyche away to his own secret place, where he protects and visits her under the cloak of darkness, so she never sees his face. Eros explains to Psyche that although he is a god, he doesn't want her to fear or revere him, but to love him as an equal. Herein, the story reveals the importance of mutuality and equality in a relationship of love.

Eventually, Psyche is coaxed (by her envious sisters) to break her vow to Eros and to attempt to see her lover in the light. So while he is sleeping, she takes a candle to bed to see his face. But the hot wax drips on his shoulder and awakens him. Sadly, Eros flies away on his white wings after telling Psyche, "Love cannot dwell with suspicion." This story conveys the invaluable lesson that trust is necessary if lovers are to remain united. In breaking their agreement to honor the mystery, Psyche attempted to know her lover through her eyes and mind, instead of allowing the *knowing* of her heart to be sufficient. Hence, in her attempt to limit and control Eros, she sacrificed everything.

Later, after Psyche is put through some seemingly impossible initiations by the goddess Venus (tests which Eros secretly helps her pass), the goddess is satisfied and allows Psyche to drink the sacred ambrosia and become immortal. Thus, Psyche is reunited with Eros, and they begin an eternal union.

Eventually, the union of Eros and Psyche (sexuality and spirituality) produces a daughter, whose name is Pleasure, suggesting that true pleasure can be attained only through the proper, healthy union of the loving soul (Psyche) with the passionate body (Eros). Furthermore, for this union to survive, it must be revered as sacred and maintain the elements of spontaneity and mystery.

DANCING TO THE UNI-VERSE (One-verse)

We all have a unique vibration and sound, a song that perfectly matches our soul. When that song is in harmony with another's, the music shared is melodic and the dance harmonious. Yet, when our vibrations are discordant, the song and rhythm will become erratic and clumsy, and the natural flow will disappear. To share the universal, sacred dance, it is necessary to accept our divinity and to realize that beneath all the many individual songs and vibrations is one ancient song encompassing all others. This ancient song calls us to share the sacred dance of the Divine.

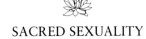

DIONYSUS–THE GOD OF ABANDON

Although the story of Dionysus might seem unfamiliar, elements of his legend are firmly embedded in modern history, religion, and psychology. Dionysus is the personification of divine ecstasy, which, in human hands, can bring either transcendent joy or madness–spiritual liberation or physical addiction. The word *ecstasy* comes from the root *ex stasis*, meaning "to stand outside oneself" (which is what happens when we have an experience that is too powerful for the body to contain).

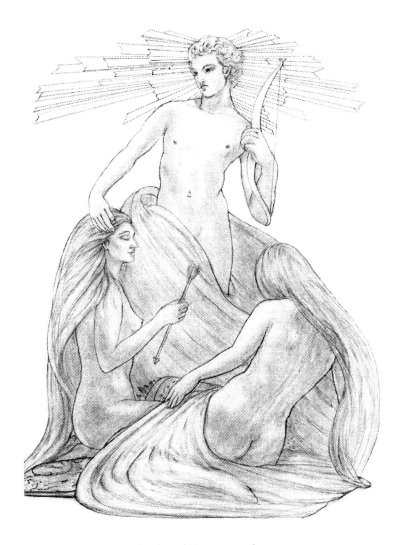

Greek god Dionysus and consorts

Dionysus is often referred to as the god of abandon, the god of ecstasy or the god of the *vine*, meaning "wine," but not "drunkenness," as often portrayed. In fact, drunkenness was not permitted at ancient Dionysian gatherings, since it was believed that one had to maintain conscious awareness to avoid being possessed by negative spirits while in such a vulnerable and open state.

Dionysus represents the ecstasy of the senses and the sensuous world and is therefore the antithesis of the intellectual thought processes. Ancient civilizations honored Dionysus by many names and in diverse forms. In fact, the practice of the *orgy* was originally a ritual honoring the god Dionysus–the god of liberation and abandon. The theatre is said to also have originated as one of the Dionysian rituals.

Since he represented the awakening of the earth, the Christians turned the youthful, androgynous, and beautiful Dionysus into a goat image, depicted with what they perceived as the face of the devil. Yet, paradoxically, many churches still practice Dionysian rituals. In fact, there are numerous parallels between Dionysus and Jesus–making Jesus a living embodiment of Dionysus. Both are sons of Divine Fathers and mortal, virgin mothers. The mothers of both are said to have ascended to Heaven. The father of Dionysus is Zeus (sometimes called *Dias-Pitar*, meaning "God, the father"), while that of Jesus is referred to as "the Father, God." Both beings are said to have visited hell, or the underworld, and both Dionysus and Jesus were hailed as "King of Kings."

Additionally, Dionysus and Jesus both die and are reborn, becoming symbols of transformation. Afterwards, Dionysus ascends to Olympus and Jesus, to Heaven, while both sit at the right hand of God. The name *Dionysus* means "son of God," while Jesus was called the "son of God."

Dionysus and Jesus both suffered at the hands of local authorities and were said to have mingled with men and women of questionable character and low repute. Also, both show a disregard for the established modes of worship.

Given all the similarities between Dionysus and Jesus, it becomes clear that both beings personify the living Christ, one as a mythological archetype and the other as a living incarnation. Dionysus is the male archetype of Christ consciousness expressed in sensual form just as Mary Magdalene is for the female.

PARADISE LOST

The English poet John Milton reveals incredible insights into the role and higher purpose of sexual encounters. In *Paradise Lost*, he depicts a conversation between Adam and the Archangel Raphael. Here, Adam shares his perplexing attraction for Eve as follows:

"To love thou blam'st me not, for love thou say'st
Leads up to heav'n, is both the way and guide;
Bear with me then, if lawful what I ask:
Love not the heav'nly spirits, and how their love
Express they, by looks only, or do they mix
Irradiance, virtual or immediate touch?"
To whom the Angel, with a smile that glowed
Celestial rosy red, love's proper hue,
Answered: "Let it suffice thee that thou know'st
Us happy, and without love no happiness.
Whatever pure thou in the body enjoy'st
(And pure thou wert created) we enjoy
In eminence, and obstacle find none
Of membrane, joint, or limb..."

In this poem, Milton touches upon some of the themes of Genesis I and II. He implies that it *is* possible for human partnerships to be blessed with love; that the body was created pure; that sexual intercourse is pure and undefiled as long as the soul and body are properly connected to their Divine Source; and that human sexual love is a reflection of a greater Love Divine. Milton also implies that although the angels have a higher vibrational presence, they still enjoy some form of passionate expression. He further indicates that despite the higher form of angelic interaction, the angels themselves do not hold a judgment for the seemingly more limited human expressions through "membranes, joints, or limbs."

THE RETURN OF THE GODDESS

There is a legend telling of a time when the gods were troubled by the appearance of a giant stone phallus (penis or lingam) that was destroying paradise. This black stone lingam was demolishing forests, homes, lakes, and mountains. The gods sent their armies to stop him but to no avail. In a moment of insight, the helpless gods remembered a great goddess whom they had formerly ignored. They humbly went to her, acknowledged her value, and said they would continue such an acknowledgement if she ended the destruction imposed by the lingam. So the goddess descended from the sky, took hold of the giant stone phallus, and slipped him deep inside of her. This act brought him such incredible pleasure that his aggression was completely dissolved.

SEXUALITY AND HOLY-DAYS

Many of humanity's holidays are actually rooted in some form of ancient sexual ritual. For example, the springtime maypole is a celebration of the lingam and fertility.

Valentine's Day originated in ancient Rome to honor the spirit of love. During valentine festivals, participants would submit their names (which were written on paper cards), and their sexual partners would be randomly selected. Thus, the custom was born of sending Valentine's Day cards to those who have captured our hearts.

The celebration known as, "Mardi Gras" was created as a festival to take place before the beginning of Lent or Ash Wednesday–a day of penance and fasting. Mardi Gras has always represented a day of wild abandon. Until the twelfth century, monks were encouraged to temporarily set aside their vows, exit their monasteries on Mardi Gras, and express all of their repressed desires. It was considered a healthy release to balance their otherwise extreme life of abstinence.

Halloween (All Hallow's Eve) was originally created to honor Dionysus, god of ecstasy. It's also believed to be the evening when the worlds of darkness and light are closest together, symbolizing the eternal dance of yin and yang or body and soul.

SHAKTI AND SHIVA

Shakti and Shiva are female and male Tantric deities representing the masculine and feminine aspects of a greater deity. Although these beings are deified, they are *both* found within all men and women. The whole universe is said to be created from the union of Shakti and Shiva.

In Hindu mythology, Shiva (man) needs Shakti (woman) to give him form, and Shakti (woman) needs Shiva (man) to give her consciousness. He can teach her wonderful things, but she can always humble him by reminding him of his limits. In this sense, the two are necessary to achieve the perfect universal dance of life.

CHAPTER 2

Modern Practices of Sacred Sex

A New Sexual Paradigm

The model of *modern* sacred sexuality has the same theme, or goal, as its predecessors, but with two primary differences. First, today's arts of sacred sex are a melting pot, or synthesis, of the more ancient practices. Second, **because of the prevalence of sexual abuse and generations of sexual repression, the future for practicing true sacred sexuality includes a greater emphasis on sexual issues and sexual healing.** This healing is necessary to make room within a person's being for a greater quantity and higher quality of energetic ecstasy.

In an age when people believe that "more is better," it's no wonder men and women obsess over shallow levels of sexual relations and feel pressured to have orgasms, or even multiple orgasms. Yet, people actually need to move in the opposite direction–slow down, relax, and heal the inhibitions, fears, and traumas causing the constrictions that prevent the fullest release and most expansive experience possible. **To experience the most profound levels of sexual ecstasy, the practitioner must be willing to release, even if only temporarily, the drive for explosive orgasms and surrender to a quest for self-discovery and healing.**

Additionally, in modern times, with so much information available on sexuality, there is a growing eclectic approach to sacred sex. People are able to pick and choose the best from all of the ancient arts of sexuality. There is also a growing use of the sexual arts for *healing*, especially for issues like sexual abuse. Consequently, as people heal, they begin to experience themselves and others differently.

The sexual healing process involves learning the difference between healthy (spiritually-centered) and unhealthy (ego-centered) sexual encounters. For example, there are numerous characteristics that differentiate an ego-centered encounter from a sacred sexual one. The former involves a search for pleasure and the fulfillment of a sense of lack, while the latter is based on sharing of expansiveness, freedom, and unconditional love. The ego-centered encounter involves judgment, control, and selfish agendas. It's motivated by the need to capture and possess a desired person (or object) who eventually becomes unfulfilling, which leads to the search for yet another person (or object). However, **in a spiritual encounter, all relationships are seen as mirrors of the self, while the heart remains open to freely express and receive love without possessiveness.** This freedom creates a feeling of inner peace and fills the body with trembling vibrations or waves of energy. Ultimately, each new (spiritually focused) sexual encounter is a fresh and loving experience that reflects the presence of the whole universe.

Love is the secret key; it opens the door to the divine. Laugh, love, be alive, dance, sing, become a hollow bamboo and let His song flow through you.

–Osho

Although no single set of guidelines for practicing sacred sexuality is right for everyone, some common principles include the following:

1. Sex is one of the most powerful manifestations of intimacy and love.
2. The most profound experience of sex begins with individual self-awareness and healing.
3. Safety is a crucial part of an intimate, ecstatic experience.
4. Foreplay is an important part of intimacy and should begin with an awareness of your partner's body and needs.
5. Sacred sexuality means paying more attention to prayer, meditation, environment, aromas, music, breathing, clothing, and intimate contact (smiling, kissing, gazing, biting, tickling, and touching).
6. Sex is not the goal in sacred sexuality–love is!
7. Orgasms are not the goal of sacred sex, so relax and enjoy *all* feelings.

8. Sacred sexuality can enhance all sensations, including orgasms.

9. When approaching an orgasm, you can choose to experience various levels of ecstatic release. There are physical orgasms (e-jaculations) and energetic orgasms (in-jaculations), as well as emotional, mental, and soul-level (total-being) orgasms.

Sex Therapy

Most sex therapists are trained counselors specializing in human sexuality and are not sex surrogates, which is another field of sexual healing. Nevertheless, because sex therapy involves a subject with such fear-based stigma, it bares the burden of controversy. For some people, sex therapy can be an invaluable way of accessing and dealing with sexual issues–potentially to a point of resolution.

A sex therapist is also an educator who is usually well informed on the subject of human sexuality. The treatment routine varies from person to person but generally includes education concerning human sexuality, as well as specific sexual exercises recommended as homework. The education and exercises are prescribed to the client and partner (if applicable) to help them reprogram their minds and bodies concerning the subject of sexuality.

Sex therapy is often sought out by individuals who suffer from such forms of sexual dysfunction as addiction and inhibitions. It is also sought out to resolve sexual issues between partners. The most common themes addressed in sex therapy are the lack of sexual arousal, the inability to reach orgasm, and the inability to orgasm during intercourse.

To treat a lack of arousal, the sex therapist usually first prescribes specific techniques for awakening the body using energy massages with as little sexual contact as possible. Then, therapy progresses to contact exercises that stimulate the entire body with touch, kisses, and massage, while focusing on each of the sensations experienced. This phase can progress to playful genital contact, but without pressure to go further. When the client is ready, he or she is urged to practice oral pleasuring to whatever degree is acceptable. The goal is to allow any fears or inhibitions to surface and pass or be re-programmed. Eventually, the client is urged to attempt intercourse with their partner, even if in limited stages.

To treat a client who is unable to have an orgasm, the sex therapist

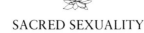

attempts to remove the client's tendency to unconsciously override the orgasmic reflex. Therapy includes accessing whatever issues are causing the mind to shut down the body's response. The treatment for such orgasmic dysfunctions includes teaching the client to relax as much as possible during sex and to recognize subtle signs of pre-orgasm. The client is urged to become aware of his or her responses if and when orgasmic sensations arise. For example, he or she might experience a tensing of muscles, a desire to leave the body, feelings of fear, and/or physical discomfort. Once these bodily clues are revealed, the therapist has a map of the terrain that needs to be explored, which is why sex therapy so often produces positive results.

To treat a client who orgasms through masturbation but not through intercourse, the sex therapist usually searches for problems in either the techniques for intercourse or the relationship itself. The treatment routine often includes working on relationship issues, as well as learning various sexual techniques. Such techniques include having the client use masturbation to build arousal as much as possible and then, just prior to reaching orgasm, begin genital thrusting with the intention of allowing the body to continue its orgasmic response. Eventually, the body becomes accustomed to the sensation of having orgasms during intercourse.

One of the most renowned sex therapists is Betty Dodson, author of *Orgasms for Two*. Betty developed masturbation workshops in the 70's and became well-known for her passion to teach women how to claim their own orgasms. To this day she holds coaching sessions in her New York apartment and offers sex education to couples. Betty notes that while it would be great for a woman to have an orgasm easily during intercourse, most women do not climax solely from vaginal penetration. So, Betty boldly teaches stimulation of the woman's sexual organs (especially the clitoris) to unlock the ability to experience orgasms.

Sexual Healing

As previously mentioned, sexual therapy is a valid technique for healing sexually related issues. However, it is but the first in at least three forms of *sexual healing*.

All forms of sexual healing are effective for balancing and healing the "root chakra" or pelvic region–areas that often hold sexual shame. Yet, despite the success of all types of sexual healing, some styles (such as sex surrogates) are still frowned upon by even the most "open-minded" healers and therapists. Therefore, getting hands-on assistance with these kinds of issues is relatively difficult, since there are very few therapists who are trained in this field and are willing to enter the realm of one of humanity's greatest taboos.

In most cases, **there are three phases of sexual healing, which should follow this order:**

1. **Sex Therapy (counseling)**
2. **Contact Therapy (hands-on)**
3. **Sacred Sexuality (such as Tantra).**

As mentioned, the most widely accepted form of sexual healing is the *first phase–sex therapy*–that actually resembles psychotherapy and mostly involves conversation, exercises and homework related to the client's particular sexual issues.

The *second phase* of sexual healing is a more radical stage, which includes the hands-on approach of *sex surrogates*. Sex surrogates are usually not licensed and are rarely acknowledged and accepted by the more mainstream professionals. Nevertheless, they play a potentially valid role in the goal of sexual healing. A trained *sex therapist* might verbally teach a man who suffers from premature ejaculation how to deal with the fears that lead to this problem. A *sexual surrogate*, on the other hand, might work with a man who suffers from premature ejaculation and show him how to prevent this problem by learning specific techniques while having sex with the therapist or surrogate. Both systems are valuable and effective, but merely take different approaches. Although it's often the case that the latter approach can lead to quicker breakthroughs, it can also stray into dangerous terrain when there may be unknown, underlying problems that a trained counselor is more prepared to deal with.

If there is any concern about potential sexual issues, inhibitions and/or abuse, the counseling phase should be experienced first. Then, the individual should move into the second, or contact phase, which might include physical bodywork, sensual massage, and even exercises in arousal.

The *third phase* of sexual healing is the practice of some type of *sacred sexuality*. Although many individuals might prefer to jump right into the third form of sexual healing (the blissful phase arising from having done thorough work in the other two stages) it's best to experience the initial two stages of sexual healing first. The initial steps of healing should reveal any personal issues concerning sexuality that need to be addressed, which, if ignored, could trigger greater trauma.

These various forms of sexual healing are not as rare as might be imagined. *Sexual healing* can be defined as "awakening a person's desire to feel alive and/or awakening the sensual self, but without the usual shame or hidden agendas." On a smaller scale, it's similar to a healer or therapist who offers a client unconditional love and acceptance, activating a deep potential for healing. It's also similar to performing a "random act of kindness" and not being attached to the outcome. In a broad sense, you offer a type of sexual healing whenever you give a compliment or appreciate someone's value, because in all such cases you are assisting to activate a person's will to live–potentially blissfully.

Ultimately, if a person can find the courage to walk through the gauntlet of sexual healing, the rewards are countless and far-reaching. While the time it takes to heal varies for each person, **the ultimate goal for all of us is to experience and integrate (1) a union with God, (2) a union within our own being (mind, body, and soul), and (3) potentially a union with partners.**

Sexual healing can assist to release trauma, restore normal sexual functions, and release unhealthy inhibitions and shame. It can also encourage self-esteem, and awaken unconditional love and self-worth–physically, emotionally, and spiritually. As we individually heal these restricting issues, we do so for all humanity.

The Role of a Sexual Partner, Healer or Therapist

Who *facilitates* sexual healing? There are counselors who specialize in this field, as well as individuals who have studied the arts of sacred sexuality. The latter group has much to offer, but a background in the psychology of trauma is highly recommended. Additionally, a friend or partner can learn some of the exercises to assist in facilitating the healing process.

There are, nonetheless, some hazards and potential pitfalls in having a friend or partner acting as the healer, rather than a therapist. If things go well, the healer often becomes the object of "transference." In this case, the client believes his or her newfound awakening is inseparably attached to the healer. On the other hand, if deep wounds are awakened, and a friend or partner is assisting the healing process, then the recipient of sexual therapy might "project" some of the hurt and rage onto the loved one. This, of course, could ruin their relationship. It is also possible to have a mixture of transference and projection.

There are precautions that can be taken to avoid the inherent pitfalls of sexual therapy. Yet, with such a taboo subject embodying so many deep issues, there are no guarantees of avoiding transference and projection. In fact, in the practice of Tantra, it's often expected that a student *will* become attracted (if not attached) to the teacher. This attraction is seen as a natural part of a student's awakening process. If treated responsibly by both parties, it can become a valuable tool to deepen their mutual vulnerability and trust.

For sexuality to reach a level worthy of being called sacred, it takes the cooperation of healthy and aware partners and healers. This healthy attitude includes unconditional love and the willingness to understand (without judging) the need for sexual healing. In other words, partners and healers must maintain an open mind and heart. Furthermore, they must develop specific skills and learn the necessary exercises for their roles as partners, healers, or therapists. Their knowledge must include (esoteric and exoteric) anatomy and physiology. Last, but not least, for partners or healers to be truly effective, they must have clear boundaries and their personal needs and issues healed (or healing).

THINGS A PARTNER OR SEXUAL HEALER SHOULD AVOID

1. Making sex (in any form) the goal of encounters.
2. Making orgasms the goal of sexual encounters.
3. Ignoring the needs of a partner or client.
4. Ignoring the issues, inhibitions, and tensions of a partner or client.
5. Disconnecting or losing the ability to remain present with a partner or client.

The Future of Sacred Sexuality

As humanity moves beyond the dogmas and stigmas that keep people imprisoned in a fear-based past, especially regarding sex, the human race will obtain a level of freedom rarely imagined. This vision of responsible love and uninhibited freedom will one day manifest for all people. This vision is at the heart of all religions and philosophies–even if they do not yet realize it. They all have the same underlying goal of returning to the All. The major difference between these various thought systems, though, is the form the journey takes. Nevertheless, out of this journey will arise a world of greater acceptance, one that honors and embraces the sacredness in all things–including sexuality.

PART III

---

*Self
Awareness*

Getting to Know You

Self-awareness means just that–you are aware of, and can focus on, *yourself*. You give top priority to the physical (Chapter 3), energetic (Chapter 4), emotional (Chapter 5), mental (Chapter 6), soul-level (Chapter 7), and spiritual (Chapter 8) aspects of your being. Furthermore, you take responsibility for your own safety and growth.

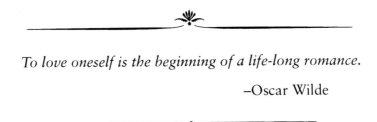

To love oneself is the beginning of a life-long romance.

–Oscar Wilde

Although the question concerning how to find the "perfect partner" is often raised, the answer lies in loving and respecting *yourself*–first. As you heal your issues and become *healthier*, you'll feel *happier* and more *attractive*. **When you feel good about yourself, it sends out positive "vibes" that are appealing to healthier partners.** Then, if and when you *do* choose to relate with another, you'll have a much better chance of developing a rewarding relationship from a solid foundation.

As you get to know yourself, you will discover personal, preconceived beliefs about love, romance, and sex. Whether conscious or not, these preconceptions definitely have an effect on your existing relationships and on those you will attract in the future. Consequently, without the necessary self-awareness, healing, and growth, **changing relationships can be like changing places of residence. You always end up having more "stuff" than you thought.**

Getting in touch with your inner self, thoughts, and beliefs paves the way for healing and blossoming into a new, more complete version of who you truly are. Whenever you do any form of inner reflecting or healing (such as through journaling), it's wise to make sure you have privacy and keep tissue nearby in case you release a few tears. To prevent your logical mind from interfering with emotions that arise, allow yourself to write spontaneously. Always begin, and end, your journaling (and any emotional process) with a prayer of dedication and surrender to God.

Since journaling and taking self-inventories are profound and insightful tools for developing self-awareness, it's worth the time to sit down to write spontaneously about the following themes:

Five things I believe about love.

1. God is Love, Love is God
2. Eternal - Divine
3. Life's currency - Self Healing, Self Sustaining
4. Love is all there is
5. Planetary evolution happens with Love

Five things I believe about sex.

1. The deepest sharing two people can have
2. Intimacy deepens a partnership
3. Love can be sex but sex doesn't equal love
4. Beautiful when shared with someone I love
5. Necessary

Five things I want from a lover.

1. Trust
2. Honesty / Integrity
3. Commitment
4. Fun
5. Delight
  Show me what you enjoy - open to learning

Five things I don't want from a lover.

1. Lack of intimacy
2. Being pounded - used like a vessel not loved & valued
3. Sex to have sex
4. Criticism
5. Body shaming

Five things that make me a good lover.

1. Curious - open
2. enthusiastic
3. enjoy pleasure, giving & receiving
4. my partner's enjoyment
5.

Five things that make me a poor lover.

1. having sex just to have sex
2. lack of interest on either side
3. lack of stimulation
4. being body shamed
5. lack of sleep, eating too much, drinking too much

Five things I remember about reaching puberty (masturbating or menstruating).

1. enjoying orgasims
2. excited to have my period - to "be a woman"
3. feeling like my breasts weren't good enough
4. no real nipple action
5. hearing sex is bad from my mom - dad saying only time they had sex they had a child.

Once you've completed your personal inventory, reflect on the results over the next several days. You may feel as though you are in "post-op" after having had emotional surgery. Yet, as you reflect, make note of any themes that stand out. For example, you may find recurring themes of guilt and shame, or your personal theme might be low self-esteem. You may discover that throughout your life others have hurt you or you may find that *you* have been the one who has most neglected or traumatized yourself. Whatever the case, if you discover any unhealthy or undesirable patterns involving your sexuality, begin making notes about how you can change these patterns. Some changes might include better physical health, a commitment to pampering and self-care, progressive counseling, or sex therapy. Such life alterations, combined with greater self-awareness, are sure to initiate positive changes in your life.

CHAPTER 3

Your Body

Getting In Touch

You can never truly give to another, what you have not accepted for yourself. So, the ability to fully give your body to a partner in sexual intimacy depends upon your ability to completely *accept* your body. In other words, if you want your partner to accept your body, you must *first* accept it yourself. You must also see yourself as loveable and worthy of acceptance.

If you don't have love for yourself, you can't be loving to others.

–Dr. Wayne Dyer

Personal Hygiene

Good hygiene is an important part of getting in touch with your body and your sexuality. There are several aspects of personal cleanliness that are invaluable, including oral, genital, and overall body hygiene. Cleanliness in all of these areas is essential in the art of sacred sexuality. It's especially important to have clean hands with well-trimmed nails. Even the slightest barb on a fingernail is capable of causing a slight cut on the sensitive tissue within the vagina or anus, which can take several days to heal.

Your body should have the scent of someone who takes care of himself or herself. You can go beyond merely having a pleasant odor and, instead, have a fragrance that is inviting to your lover.

A lack of good hygiene may result from not having been taught cleanliness in childhood. But unpleasant body odors can also be caused by diet, excessive sweat, genetics or poor health and excessive toxins in the body. If there is an issue with hygiene and you remain oblivious or careless, it can put your lover in the awkward position of telling you about it. No matter how awkward, the topic should be discussed and solutions sought and practiced.

Nutrients and Herbs

Although there are numerous constraints on what claims can be made for dietary supplements, tradition still maintains that some supplements and specific foods are enhancing to a person's sexual health. While there are many aspects of health that affect sexual performance, nothing is more important to the physical body's health than an individual's vitality and immunity, which are directly related to the health of the endocrine glands. Therefore, it's wise to pay special attention to nutrients, supplements, and a diet that nourishes the blood and immune system.

Unlike other glands, the endocrine glands (such as the pituitary, pineal, and thymus) produce hormones that are released directly into the bloodstream, sending commands to the entire body. When all the endocrine glands are in proper balance and are producing hormones at the optimum rate, the body will not age and will flourish with vitality and sexual well-being.

Despite the priority of overall health for ensuring sexual vigor, it's not uncommon for individuals to use supplements as aphrodisiacs. These stimulants (and adaptogens, which normalize secretions) are common today in organic form and/or through prescription drugs. Yet, the ideal in sacred sexuality is to maintain a balanced state of health and allow this natural vitality of being to express itself passionately with little need for "turn-on" boosters. Nevertheless, since many individuals do not maintain an optimum level of well-being, the following section lists some essential foods and supplements that enhance sexual health.

NUTRIENTS

ANTIOXIDANT VITAMINS & MINERALS–include vitamins A and C, as well as coenzyme Q10, beta carotene, and selenium. Antioxidants are found in many fresh fruits and green, leafy vegetables.

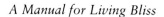

LECITHIN–indirectly adds to the production of various sex hormones.

MINERALS: CALCIUM, MAGNESIUM, & PHOSPHORUS–are a good combination for developing and maintaining healthy, sexual desire.

NIACIN–can be a powerful sexual supplement and, when taken before sex, can intensify orgasms because of an increased histamine release.

VITAMIN E–assists the blood and oxygen flow to the sex organs, which helps to maintain erection and arousal, as does the amino acid arginine.

WATER–Another important contribution to a person's optimal health and vigor is the consistent intake of large quantities of water, which flush the body of toxins and create a healthy environment for the cells.

ZINC–is good for the prostate gland and helps the male produce healthier sperm. Zinc deficiencies can contribute to prostatitis (which can add to the problem of premature ejaculation) and impotence in the male. In the female, zinc deficiency can result in insufficient vaginal lubrication. Some of the best sources of zinc are oysters and raw pumpkin seeds.

HERBS

DONG QUAI–does for a female what ginseng does for a male. It is a great tonic for healing and sexual health. Female Taoist sexual masters often recommend drinking one cup of dong quai tea per day. However, it is to be avoided if a woman is asthmatic or pregnant. Otherwise, dong quai is well known for lessening menstrual flow and increasing energy and vitality. It also tones the breasts, making them firmer.

GINSENG–is good for the metabolic rate and for increasing vitality. It acts as a tonic to the glands and nervous system (better for men than women).

SAW PALMETTO–is good for prostate problems and acts as a tonic for debility. It's also believed to alleviate some of the basic ailments of the prostate gland. Saw palmetto facilitates adequate blood flow to the prostate and penis and prevents complications with the urethra during aging.

YOHIMBE–is considered a potent sexual supplement. It is said to expand blood vessels in the extremities of the body (including the genitals) and enhance erections.

Hormones

There are hundreds of hormones in the human body, but only a few are directly related to sexual health. The word *hormone* comes from the Greek phrase "to excite." Most hormones are produced in the endocrine glands–the pituitary being the master gland. The two best-known *sexual* hormones are estrogen (found in greater amounts in women) and testosterone (found in greater amounts in men).

From a physiological perspective, during romantic relationships, the pituitary gland activates and commands several of the body's endocrine glands to secrete various "love" hormones. One such hormone is pheny-lethylamine (PEA), which is said to create a subtle state of euphoria wherein physical pain decreases, depression disappears, and we feel more alive. Experienced in the early stage of a romantic relationship, this hormonal euphoria is sometimes misinterpreted as "true love" but has been proven to last for only about six months. When this euphoria fades, all of our problems return, and we think love has worn off. Incidentally, there is PEA in chocolate.

DHEA is found in high concentrations in both males and females. DHEA is primarily produced in the adrenals but is also created in the ovaries and testicles. DHEA strengthens the immune system, acts as an antidepressant, and is believed to boost the production of some sexual hormones.

ESTROGEN represents the *yin* principle and in the woman is created mostly in the ovaries. Estrogen lubricates the vagina, strengthens the tissue of the sexual organs, and encourages changes in the uterus during menstruation. Estrogen is a neurologic exciter that enhances the limbic appreciation centers of the brain, making sensations more intense.

OXYTOCIN is produced in the hypothalamus but is stored in the pituitary gland. Oxytocin promotes greater sensitivity in the skin, creates loving and sensuous feelings, awakens a desire for touch, and stimulates nurturing love. Oxytocin also acts as a contractive hormone for the uterus and the muscle in the prostate. The muscular "tightness" (or contraction) felt with orgasm is believed to be due to this hormone.

PHEROMONES are actually *not* hormones but are still relevant for evoking sexual response. Pheromones are in highest concentration in such bodily secretions as sweat, saliva, and sexual fluids.

PROGESTERONE is used to raise testosterone levels, has a slightly calming effect, and eases menstrual cramps.

TESTOSTERONE represents the yang principle and is created mostly in the testicles and adrenals. Testosterone stimulates the desire for sex, increases assertiveness and competitiveness, and strengthens thinking processes.

Celibacy and the Spiritual Path

The issue of celibacy surfaces at some point for nearly every student who embarks on the spiritual path. Yet, a common misconception exists concerning the definition of *celibacy*. Celibacy, by its true definition, involves making a personal choice to *completely* abstain from sex (including masturbation). During this period of abstinence, sexual energy is consciously channeled throughout the body for a higher purpose.

There are potentially both positive and negative effects from practicing celibacy. The positive effects include developing self-discipline and using sexual energy to enhance health and vitality. The negative effects include the possibility of experiencing personal frustration and depression. It's no secret that some sexual desires kept repressed, or suppressed, can cause physical, emotional, and anxiety-related disorders. The physical body's natural biological needs must be met. In fact, the arousal of the reproductive organs without expression can cause the cells within the sexual glands to disintegrate. It can also adversely affect the entire nervous system. These negative results can be transformed with the proper use of sexual exercises, such as those found in this book.

Masturbation

There are both positive and negative aspects to masturbation, or self-pleasuring. With the proper focus and intent, self-pleasuring is an act of self-love. It is an effective method for awakening one's physical level of consciousness, as well as for relaxing, learning, exploring, and awakening repressed parts of the sexual anatomy. When used properly, self-stimulation can ignite powerful surges that awaken energetic ecstasy. Also, for individuals who have issues with self-love, pleasuring themselves can be a means of developing self-acceptance. Unfortunately, because of the issues surrounding sexuality, self-pleasuring was not deemed "normal" behavior by the A.M.A. until the early 1970's.

Self-pleasuring also has its darker, addictive side. Although it is quite natural for a person to stimulate and explore his or her own body, masturbation has become a rampant addiction (repetitive attempts to fill a perceived void) for many men and a growing one for women. Men have gained a reputation for browsing the Internet for porn sights to appease their need for a sexual release. Women, on the other hand, are becoming accustomed to reaching for vibrators to assist their pleasuring. But if vibrators are used excessively, they can result in women's bodies refusing to respond to any other form of stimulation, such as touch or intercourse. This *dependency* on a mechanical device is counterproductive to the goals of intimacy and sacred sexuality.

When Edgar Cayce, the world's greatest modern seer, was asked about the effects of masturbation, his replies varied between *advantageous* and *detrimental*. For some clients, he stated that masturbation was a healthy practice. Yet for others, he claimed it was harmful. Cayce said that if masturbation became an obsession, it was better to redirect such thoughts and actions toward more constructive things. Still, he suggested that when a person was organically aroused, he or she should do something with the energy; otherwise, cells within the sexual glands would be destroyed. Yet the same advice did not apply for a sexual addict who constantly self-stimulates, which was said to result in the depletion of vitality. Cayce told one gentleman that the over-stimulation of his genital system was causing him nervous digestion and the depletion of his heart's energy. Cayce's insights seem to suggest that **self-pleasuring can be a form of self-love or self-abuse, depending on the focus of intent underlying the act.** The ancient practitioners of sacred sexuality clearly agree.

Impotence

The word *impotence* has different meanings when applied to men and women. For women, it can refer to a case of infertility. For men, impotence can refer to the inability to have or maintain an erection. An erectile problem is experienced by most men at some point in their lives, especially during late middle age. But difficulty in maintaining an erection often results from depleted vitality, rather than advanced age.

Taoist sexual practitioners recommend increasing the body's reserve of vitality as a means of balancing and improving health. Once normal

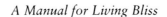
erections are reestablished (or before the problem with erection occurs) men should practice sex without ejaculation.

Both men and women depend on their inner vitality to keep their immune systems functioning at an optimum level and their health at its peak. This vitality can be charged and increased with the proper use of the sexual forces.

For both men and women, impotence can also refer to the inability to reach a climax, or orgasm. This difficulty is usually rooted in emotional issues, more so than physical or energetic problems. It most commonly has to do with fear of losing control, anxiety over vulnerability, or issues of guilt or shame. All of these issues can be healed through counseling or sex therapy.

Anatomy 101

A basic, elementary way of differentiating a male from a female in nearly every species is by checking the genitals because our eyes tell us there is such an obvious distinction between the sexes. Yet, contrary to what most people believe, the sexual anatomy of a male and a female is actually very similar, despite having *some* differences.

He who knows the truth of the body can then know the truth of the universe.

–Rat Nas Tantra

Essentially we all originate as androgynous (combined male *and* female) beings and energetically remain such throughout our lives. Although not evident to the eyes, this fact remains true. We all have a right (feminine, creative) lobe of the brain and a left (masculine, logical). We all have yin (feminine) and yang (masculine) meridians flowing through our bodies. Our genitals are merely the outer manifestations of our primary physical expressions as either predominately male or female. During the earliest stages of fetal development, there is no known sexual differentiation between the two genders. Sexual differentiation does not become apparent until the fetus is several weeks old.

During fetal development, the reproductive system begins as a tiny mass that resembles an ice cream cone with a round knob at the top and a pillar-like base, or shaft, below. The rounded top morphs into the head of either the clitoris or penis. The shaft then splits down the middle becoming the two labia minora of the vagina or remains intact as the two chambers of the corpora cavernosa within the penis.

After the differentiation becomes clear, the masculine and feminine bodies develop in favor of their specific gender. The male (being root-chakra based) projects sexual anatomy (his penis) from his groin. The female (being heart-chakra based) projects sexual anatomy (her breasts) from her heart. These seemingly opposite projections symbolically suggest that a man is given the key (his penis) to penetrate and unlock a woman's body, and a woman is given the key (her breast) to penetrate and unlock a man's heart.

Each major part of the human sexual anatomy of one gender is analogous to the anatomy of the opposite gender. For example, a clitoris is merely a female's version of a penis, and a man's prostate is the male's version of a G-spot. Examples of the anatomical parallels include:

FEMALE	MALE
Clitoris	Head of Penis
Clitoral Hood	Foreskin of Penis
Clitoral Legs	Legs of Corpora Cavernosa
G-spot	Prostate
Lips Majora	Scrotum
Lips Minora	Shaft of Penis
Ovaries	Testicles
Vaginal canal	Skin of Penis Shaft
Vestibular Bulb	Bulb or Base of the Penis

Although this understanding of the male and female anatomies and insight into the mutual importance of each gender are common knowledge to those who practice sacred sexuality, they are usually unknown to most.

To prevent any confusion over varying terminology, this chapter will generally refer to the male and female sexual anatomy by the traditional names of *penis* and *vagina*.

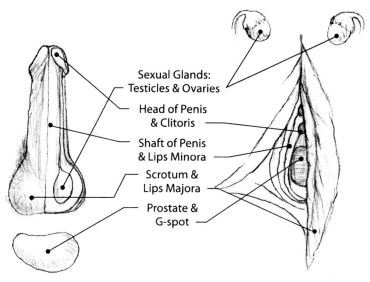

Sexual Glands:
Testicles & Ovaries

Head of Penis
& Clitoris

Shaft of Penis
& Lips Minora

Scrotum &
Lips Majora

Prostate &
G-spot

Anatomical parallels between a male and female

THE FEMALE

The female sexual organs are divided into two groups. The *external* genitalia, which is known as the "vulva," and the *internal* cavity, commonly called the "vagina," which means "sheath" or "purse" (a pouch in which to place something).

I. THE OUTSIDE (Vulva)

The anatomy of the vulva (as described in this book) includes all visible parts of the genitalia including the *pubic mound*, the *lips majora*, and the *clitoris*.

THE PUBIC MOUND (Mons) is a mound of padding, or fatty tissue, with a covering of pubic hair. This mound of extra padding covers the "pubic bone" to protect it from injury during sexual thrusting.

THE LABIA MAJORA (Outer, Major Lips) are the two swollen-like mounds on each side of the vaginal opening. The labia majora are primarily two folds of skin containing, fatty tissue, sweat glands, blood vessels, and nerve endings. These folds of adipose tissue, which can engorge with arousal or manual stimulation, are the female's version of the male scrotum. These mounds act as an enclosure for the inner lips and other, more sensitive, portions of the inner vagina.

THE CLITORIS (nature's Rubik's Cube), which means "key" in Greek,

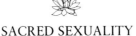
has only one known function–arousing pleasure. The head and shaft portion of the clitoris is an average of about one inch long and believed to have eight thousand nerve endings, the highest concentration in the body. A penis has about half as many nerve endings. The clitoris is basically a miniature penis with the same three parts: the head (or glans), the body (or shaft), and the legs (or crura). The clitoris is only partly an external organ, as only the head (glans) and a portion of the shaft are actually visible. Most of its length is buried beneath the surface of the body. The full clitoris (from its head to the end of its legs) looks like a wishbone.

The clitoris is like a flower. The head is the bud, the shaft is the stem, and legs are the roots. The stem passes from the head, through the shaft and into the legs of the clitoris. The clitoris varies slightly in size from one woman to the next. When stimulated, a clitoris (like a penis) can engorge to two or three times its flaccid size. A clitoris is capable of being aroused and feeling sensation without any actual physical contact.

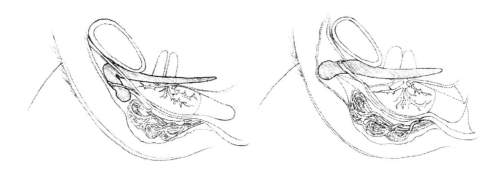

Female clitoris in the limp and erect stages

The clitoris is sharply bent slightly below the head. The head bows forward towards the opening of the vagina until it becomes erect, at which point it stands at attention. When a woman is fully aroused, her clitoris seems to retract, or shrink, which is sometimes related to fear and emotional issues. But usually, this retraction is a way for the clitoris to become cocked and ready to fire. As arousal continues, the woman's clitoral hood swells, further hiding the clitoral head.

Unlike the clitoris, a stimulated penis engorges and traps the blood within its chambers until an orgasm has passed. But since the clitoris lacks the "lock and load" tendency of the penis, it fills and empties its blood flow continually, allowing it to reach orgasm again and again. This filling and emptying of blood also accounts for the tendency of the clitoris to swell and appear, only to disappear again–even without having an orgasm.

The Clitoral Head has the highest concentration of pleasure nerve endings in the body. Still, as many men and women have discovered, it is quite elusive and can remain hidden under its hood. The clitoral head is the object of most physical stimulation for women, as it usually triggers the quickest orgasms and sexual excitation.

Unfortunately, each year millions of young girls (and some women) have a portion of their clitoris (usually the head) removed in the name of culture and religion. This practice, known as a clitoridectomy, is one of a few surgical procedures aimed at the removal of a portion of the female genitalia.

The Shaft connects the glans (head) to the crura (legs) of the clitoris. The head is the most sensitive part of the clitoris, but the shaft and roots are also responsive to stimulation and pleasuring–finding them is another story. Like the penis, the clitoris has erectile structures (the corpora cavernosa) that make up a major portion of the shaft. The two crura, which divide into two separate "legs" at the base of the clitoris, engorge with blood during stimulation, resulting in an erection of the clitoris.

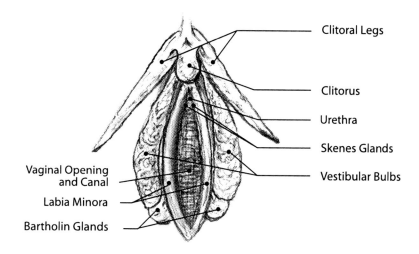

Detailed drawing of the exposed female sexual anatomy

The Clitoral Legs (crura) originate as the shaft of the clitoris but divide into two tail-lie appendages, approximately three to four inches long. They are analogous to the corpus cavernosum of the penis. Although the clitoral legs are not visible, they can be contacted by rubbing along the underside of the pelvic bone (just below the pubic bone) and run downward, along either side of the vaginal opening and beneath the lips minora.

The Clitoral Hood is not actually a part of the clitoris but is vital enough to the clitoris to mention here. The clitoral hood is a thin fold of skin that surrounds the clitoris and acts as a hood, or cover, but is slightly mobile and loose fitting. Some women find the clitoris too sensitive to be touched directly. In such cases, try stimulating the clitoris through the hood.

II. THE INSIDE (Vagina)

The internal female sexual organs are all housed within the pelvic cavity. The primary internal sexual anatomy of a woman includes the *labia minora*, *vestibular bulbs*, the *G-spot*, the *vaginal canal*, and the *uterus* and *ovaries*.

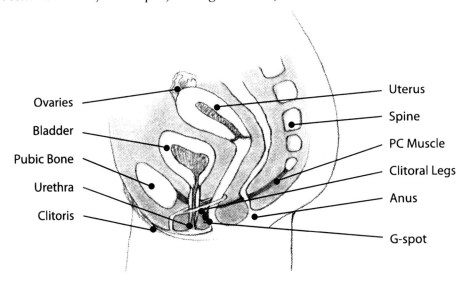

Side view of the female sexual anatomy

The vaginal canal is an energetic cauldron whose magic is best activated by focusing on love, being present with your lover, and making the proper contact with and stimulation of her other sensual triggers, such as the breasts, clitoris, G-spot, and anus. The magical ingredients of this sacred, energetic cauldron respond best when cooked slowly and left on simmer. This simmering activates energy within the vagina that can send powerful surges or gentle waves upward through a woman's body. It may take a while for a woman to become accustomed to this energetic surge within her body, especially if she has grown used to clitoral stimulation.

The Valley spirit never dies. It is named the mysterious female. And the doorway of the mysterious female is the base from which heaven and earth sprang. It is there, within us all the while; draw upon it as you will, it never runs dry.

—*Tao-Te Ching*

If a woman feels energy building within her vagina and starts contracting her pelvic muscles or excessively moving her pelvis, her vagina will attempt to reach for an orgasm, similar to a man's. At such times, her vagina creates an intense swirling energy that grips the man's penis, as if grabbing it, shaking it, and saying, "give me my orgasm." This is one of many reasons why it is better for a woman to learn to relax through all temptations to contract her pelvic muscles when becoming aroused or near orgasm.

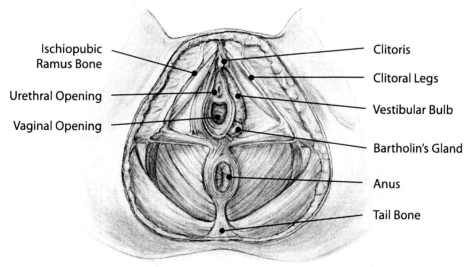

Exposed female muscles and genitals

THE LABIA MINORA (inner, minor lips) are on each side of a woman's vaginal opening and become engorged when stimulated. The labia minora

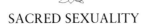

come in a variety of shapes and sizes. They extend upward from the bottom to the top of the vaginal opening. It is near the clitoris that the labia minora join in two places: first, above the clitoris (forming the clitoral hood) and, second, just below the clitoris (forming the sensitive frenulum). The inner labia can be gently separated to expose the clitoris. When the labia are separated, the vaginal opening (known as the introitus), composed of shiny tissue, is also exposed, as is the tip of the urinary (urethral) opening, located between the vaginal opening and the clitoris.

The inner lips do not contain hair follicles but are rich with sweat glands, sebaceous scent glands, blood vessels, and nerves. The inner lips do not have the fatty tissue of the outer lips, which allows them to function as erectile tissue during intercourse.

THE VESTIBULAR BULBS are analogous to both the male's corpus spongiosum and the bulb of his penis. These two objects of erectile tissue are hidden beneath the lips minora and run along each side of the vaginal opening, starting from the clitoris. Covered with a mass of coiled blood vessels, the vestibular bulbs are erectile and therefore swell with sexual arousal. They also transfer blood to and from the clitoral shaft and are, in fact, closely related to the clitoris and its response. At the lower portion of the vestibular bulbs (towards the lower part of the vaginal opening) are the vestibular glands (or Bartholin glands), which secrete fluid for vaginal lubrication and during female ejaculations.

THE G-SPOT, the female equivalent of the male prostate gland, was named after the doctor who is reported to have "discovered" it, Dr. Ernst von Grafenberg. It's ironic, to say the least, that a doctor of the twentieth century should place his name on a part of the female anatomy that was known and explored in ancient sexual manuscripts thousands of years ago. So modern practitioners of sacred sexuality changed the meaning of the abbreviation "G" to the "goddess-spot." The ancients actually referred to it as the "sacred spot."

The G-spot, by any name, is actually not a "spot" at all, but a region that surrounds the urethra as it passes along the ceiling of the vagina. It's an area within the vaginal canal filled with *nerves* that respond to arousal. The paraurethral (Skene's) *glands* that create vaginal orgasm and ejaculation with proper stimulation are a part of the G-spot region located on the roof of the vagina, just an inch or so from the vaginal opening.

Although the surrounding vaginal canal lacks nerve endings, the G-spot is caressed by the nerves that bring pleasure to the clitoris. Since the vaginal wall contains few nerve receptors for touch and pleasure, stimulation of the G-spot (manually or through intercourse) helps to create a *"vaginal* orgasm," or an orgasm without stimulation of the clitoris. There is also a nerve connection from the G-spot to the bladder, which is one of the primary reasons for the sensation to urinate when the G-spot is stimulated.

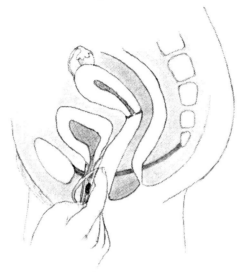

Locating the G-spot

To find the G-spot, insert one or two fingers into the vagina and stroke or massage the spongy tissue at the roof of the vagina. The G-spot swells when stimulated and feels similar to the rough or bumpy section on the roof of the mouth. Since the urethral canal runs through the center of the vagina's roof, stroking can add to the sensation to urinate. This sensation can be avoided by not massaging directly in the center of the vaginal canal. Strangely enough, even though the G-spot can be felt *and* its stimulation can trigger a unique form of orgasm, many medical researchers and manuals do not acknowledge its existence–even in today's "modern" age.

The G-spot is the place where women psychically store their cellular memories of sexual issues and abuses. Therefore, massaging this area can sometimes result in the release of old wounds. If cellular memories and sexual wounds are accessed therapeutically, the results can be profound. But, if awakened without proper knowledge and experience, the results can sometimes be overwhelming to either or both partners. Bodily memories can surface that result in various forms of emotional release and energetic discharges. Or, more rarely, the woman can go into minor levels of shock. Even so, releasing any stored trauma or memories is important for healing.

One technique for releasing trauma or stored memories is for a woman (or her partner) to massage the G-spot with healing intent, by consciously sending loving energy to this area. During a healing session, there should be no attempt to produce a particular sexual response. While the G spot is gently and slowly being massaged, the woman should notice any and all sensations experienced in that area. There are three potential sensations that can arise: numbness, pain, and/or pleasure. If a woman begins healing of the G-spot, she often experiences all three of these sensations. She may have one sensation more than the others but it is not uncommon to feel all three during each healing session. The numb and painful sensations may pass in one session or over a period of months. Whatever the case, be patient and never rush.

THE VAGINAL CANAL is a musculomembranous canal that connects the uterus to the external genitalia. It measures an average of four inches, and its walls are heavily folded, allowing it to expand during intercourse or childbirth. When a woman becomes genitally aroused, her vaginal wall usually balloons outward. By consciously pushing her vaginal muscles down, she collapses this balloon effect, resulting in a tighter, more stimulating fit for the penis during intercourse.

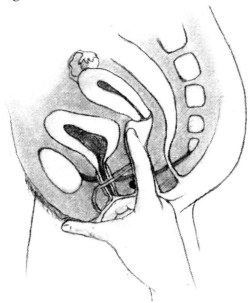

Stimulating the vaginal canal

EXERCISE:

Healing with a Mineral Egg

The following exercise is for healing psychic and emotional wounds within the uterus and vaginal canal. This egg exercise can draw out stored, negative energy and memories. It involves inserting a smooth, polished mineral egg (such as quartz crystal) into your vaginal canal. These eggs can be purchase at most rock and gem shows or at "New Age" bookstores.

Choose a mineral egg, such as crystal, amethyst or rose quartz, preferably with a hole drilled through one end. Most of the sizes that stores carry will work fine. Before beginning, make sure you have cleansed your egg by soaking it in sea salt for several hours and by simmering it in water for about ten minutes—being careful not to crack or break it through overheating. Once the egg is cleaned and purified, tie a piece of floss through the end so the egg can be removed like a tampon. If your egg cannot be tied with floss, just make sure you feel comfortable placing it inside while knowing that you will have to use your vaginal muscles to force it back out.

1. Remove all of your clothes except for your underpants, as they may be needed to catch the egg if it slips from the vagina.

2. Stand with your feet at shoulders' width apart and knees unlocked. After rubbing a little lubrication on the egg, insert it into your vaginal canal.

3. Place your hands over your heart center while breathing slowly and deeply.

4. After five or ten minutes of centering, slide the fingertips of one hand down to your lower abdomen as if brushing energy downward. Do this several times. Begin visualizing energy moving down into your uterus and vagina.

5. Once you feel a distinct connection between your heart and vaginal canal, begin using your vaginal muscles to move the egg further up into the canal on each deep inhalation. Do nothing except relax on the exhale.

6. When the egg feels as though it has entered far enough, spend five to ten minutes rubbing your lower abdomen while visualizing the egg absorbing negative energy from your body.

7. Next, begin pushing the egg downward with each deep exhalation until it exits or is close enough to be pulled out.

8. When you are finished, do some grounding exercises. Then soak your egg overnight in sea salt.

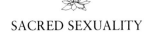
THE UTERUS is, in Taoist sexual practices, referred to as "The Heavenly Palace." The uterus is depicted as "heavenly" because of its abode–hovering above the other sexual organs–and because of its purpose, which is to be a heavenly home for the developing fetus prior to entering the earth plane.

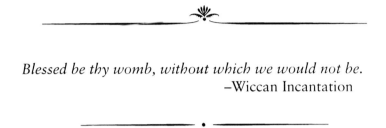

Blessed be thy womb, without which we would not be.
–Wiccan Incantation

The uterus, or womb, is a muscular organ located behind, and slightly above, the bladder. Shaped like an upside down pear, the uterus is, on average, three inches in length and two inches at its widest portion. During menstruation, the lining of the uterus (known as the endometrium) increases in thickness to receive and nourish a fertilized egg. If a fertilized egg attaches to the lining, the uterus expands and becomes more muscular to contain the growing baby. These muscles will later be used to contract and push the baby out of the womb during birth. When a fertilized egg does not arrive, the lining breaks down and is released from the uterus and out of the vagina through menstruation.

The uterus is typically overlooked as part of the sexual anatomy. This neglect results primarily from its lack of exposure to direct physical stimulation and from a lack of understanding concerning how it can be energetically activated.

The uterus is such a vital part of the female sexual anatomy that it is a primary storehouse for memories from physical, emotional, and psychic sexual abuse. By nature, the uterus opens to receive the male's semen. A woman willingly opens to receive the male because she unconsciously seeks to be filled, preferably in her heart, but she'll settle for her womb. Because of her willingness to settle, she often ends up absorbing a great deal of unhealthy energy from the male.

Every woman should connect and share healing time on a regular basis with her uterus. Some of this healing can be done through energy work, prayer, journaling and/or visualization. A woman can have a dialog with her uterus, allowing it to speak about its condition–good or ill. Her uterus might speak of being wounded, angry or afraid. Or it might express being safe, loved or nurtured.

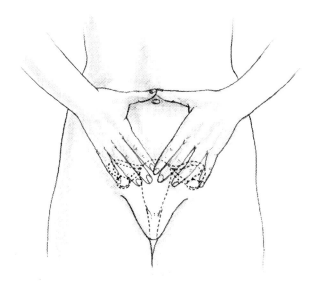

Locating the female ovaries and uterus

Doing healing energy work on the uterus and ovaries is a subtle and complicated process, difficult to describe and in need of a very sensitive, intuitive healer. Reiki is an excellent method for sending love into either the uterus or the ovaries.

EXERCISE:
Spiritual Pregnancy

A woman's desire to love and be loved is often misinterpreted by her body as the urge to be filled with a child whom she can love. As a result, a woman who has never been pregnant may feel incomplete. Whether or not a woman ever becomes physically pregnant, all women should regularly fill their uteruses with light–becoming pregnant with love and birthing that love every day.

1. Sit comfortably in a chair or at the head of your bed.
2. Close your eyes and do a few minutes of deep, centering breathing.
3. Use your fingertips to lightly massage/stimulate around your nipples.

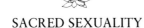
4. Use your fingertips to lightly massage/stimulate your inner thighs (from knees to groin).

5. When you are aware of a clear, heightened state of arousal, allow moans to emit from your belly and through your throat center.

6. Then visualize light and energy being drawn up into your vaginal canal from the ethers surrounding you and then into your uterus and ovaries (or where they would be if they have been removed).

7. Trap the energy there and use one hand (or both) to make gentle spirals on your tummy. Visualize a ball of light in your uterus. It's your baby, a creation of yours that can become anything you want.

8. Give your baby an identity, not a name per se but a concept. Identify it as something you want to bring into your life, such as prosperity or self-worth.

9. Each morning and evening, before you rise or prepare for sleep, rub your tummy, visualize this ball of light, and acknowledge its identity. Then affirm that you have become immaculately impregnated with this gift from God. Also affirm that you are now prepared for its birth into your life.

THE OVARIES, like the uterus, are usually overlooked as a part of the sexual anatomy. Yet, since the ovaries generate the eggs to create a human being, they possess a great deal of power. The ovaries also produce hormones, such as estrogen, which influences a female's sexual development. In effect, the ovaries are storehouses for a woman's sexual power and development. For this reason, Taoists have specific exercises to tone and warm the ovaries.

The exact location of the ovaries varies slightly from woman to woman. In general, if you place your hands flat on your abdomen, with the heel of your hands resting on the front of your hip bones, the tips of your thumbs meeting at your navel, and your fingers angled toward your pubic bone, your fingers should be resting over the area of your ovaries.

EXERCISE:
Ovary Massage

Ovarian massage is a highly effective method for accessing a woman's creative, sexual power and transforming it into useable life-force. This exercise channels and directs a woman's sexual energy throughout her entire body. It also balances and regulates her hormones and her menstrual cycle.

1. Stand or sit comfortably and practice some slow, deep abdominal breaths.
2. Rub your hands together to warm them and activate their sensitivity to energy.
3. Place one hand on each of your ovaries (or where they would be if they have been removed).
4. Press your fingertips in slightly to contact the ovaries and begin massaging the area over the ovaries a few dozen times in a circular motion. Then repeat in the opposite direction.
5. As the energy within the ovaries becomes activated, the ovaries will start to feel warm.
6. Next, visualize the energy moving through the fallopian tubes and into the uterus.
7. Now keep your fingers resting on the ovaries as you visualize and feel the energy from the ovaries creating a glowing, warm, healing sensation throughout the lower abdomen.
8. Conclude by taking several slow deep breaths as you use your fingertips to stroke the energy from the abdomen and draw it to all parts of the body.

THE MALE

Like the female anatomy, the male sexual organs can be divided into two groups. The *external* portion is known as the *scrotum* and *penis*. The *internal* portion includes the *testicles* and *prostate gland*.

I. THE OUTSIDE (Scrotum and Penis)

The anatomy of a male (as described in this book) encompasses all visible parts of the genitalia including the outer skin of the *scrotum* and the primary anatomy of the *penis* with its internal parts.

The male penis is known in Sanskrit by other names, including *lingam* (meaning "Wand of Light") and *vajra* (meaning "Thunderbolt"). This should help to illustrate the power and splendor of the penis. Much like a dragon, when asleep, it's fairly sedate. Yet when awake, the penis becomes a symbol of virility and strength. A woman's yoni may be a sacred cauldron, but the man has the wand that stirs and ignites the magic.

THE SCROTUM is the sack that hangs below the penis. It contains the male sexual glands known as the testes, or testicles, the male version of the female's ovaries. During fetal development, the male testicles reside up in the abdominal cavity, similar to a female's ovaries, and gradually descend into the scrotum. The scrotum usually hangs loosely from the body, but there are times when it shrivels up tightly. Such moments include cold weather, fear or during an approaching orgasm.

From the outside, the scrotum looks like only one single part. But internally, it is divided into two parts (left and right), each containing one testicle. The left testicle hangs a little lower than the right, preventing excessive bumping between the testicles.

THE PENIS in its flaccid, non-erect, state averages three inches long and one-and-a-half inches in diameter. The average erect penis is between five and six inches. The longer a penis is when it's flaccid, the less it will grow to reach an erection. An erection is the result of blood engorging tiny caverns, or sinuses, within three chambers that run the length of the penis. The amount of blood that flows into an erection is nearly ten times that which is present before the erection. An erection is usually the result of sexual stimulation but can also occur at other times, such as during sleep.

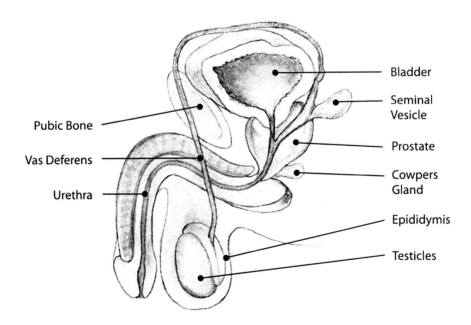

Side view of the male sexual anatomy

Like a woman's clitoris (her version of a penis), a man's penis divides into three parts: the head (or glans), the body (or shaft), and the legs (or crura). Also, like a clitoris, the penis is only partly exposed, with just the head and most of the shaft being visible. The roots or legs of the penis are inside the man's pelvic cavity.

The penis also has a *base*, which extends internally into the pelvic cavity. The male corpus spongiosum runs from the head of the penis down to the base, which terminates at the bulb below the pubic bone and is energetically connected to the prostate.

The bulb becomes rigid and enlarged during arousal, almost filling the entire space between the surrounding pelvic bones. When enlarged, the bulb also presses downward on the testicles. The bulb of the penis is analogous to the vestibular bulbs of the female. In fact, there is a small groove at the end of the bulb, known as the embryonic groove. The presence of this groove reveals that in embryonic development, there were once two bulbs (as in the female) that eventually fused together to form a single bulb.

The Head of the penis is covered with a foreskin unless the penis has been circumcised, in which case, the head is fully exposed. But even if the foreskin has not been removed, the head of the penis usually penetrates beyond the extra skin during an erection. Just below the head of the penis and on the underside, is the most sensitive part of the male sexual anatomy–the frenulum.

The Shaft of the penis is the longest portion. The shaft connects the head to the base and legs of the penis. Inside the shaft is the urethra, the long slender tube within the penis, used for urination and ejaculation. The penis shaft consists of nerves, fibrous tissue, blood vessels, and three chambers of spongy tissue.

These three chambers fill with blood during an erection, causing the hardening of the penis. Two of the three chambers are called "corpora cavernosa," meaning cavernous bodies. The third chamber is called "corpus spongiosum," meaning spongy body. The two cavernous bodies run along the sides of the penis and help to increase its thickness and hardness during erection. The spongy body begins in the penile head (helping it to enlarge) and runs along the underside of the penis until it roots itself in the bulb-like fixture at the base of the penis. These spongy chambers have numerous hollow cavities richly supplied with blood vessels.

The Roots or Legs of the penis extend internally into the pelvic cavity, as do the legs of a woman's clitoris. The two corpora cavernosa of the penis's shaft divide and attach to the underside of the man's pelvic bones (below the pubic bone), much like the two clitoral legs in a woman. These legs are often dense and hard with muscular armoring resulting from sexual fears and inhibitions. With deep, yet sensitive, massaging, they can be healed, softened, and re-sensitized for greater sensitivity and pleasure.

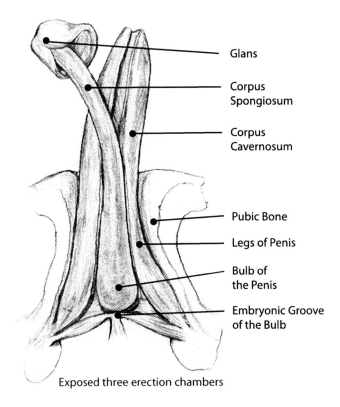

Glans

Corpus Spongiosum

Corpus Cavernosum

Pubic Bone

Legs of Penis

Bulb of the Penis

Embryonic Groove of the Bulb

Exposed three erection chambers

EXERCISE:

Penis Enlargement

It is generally assumed that, other than using medicine or surgery, the size of a penis cannot be altered. This, however, is not the case. As previously mentioned, the shaft of the penis is mostly composed of three chambers that fill with blood during arousal. These chambers are made of soft, flexible tissue, which can be stretched or lengthened. If the chambers are stretched, there is more room within their empty spaces, which means more room for blood during an erection. The more blood that fills the penis, the larger and harder the erection. The following exercise stretches the chambers within the penis thus enlarging the penis and its erection. It should be practiced a few days per week for several weeks. If there is ever excessive discomfort, you should stop the exercise.

1. Stand or sit comfortably.
2. Apply a lubricant that will work well for you. It must keep your skin from becoming irritated but must not cause your hand to slip too easily. Rub the lubricant on and create a mild erection.
3. Gently, but securely, grip around the base of your penis using the thumb and index finger of one hand.
4. With the thumb and index finger of your other hand, grip just below the head of the penis, as you inhale deeply.
5. Exhale with a deep, "huh," sound as you slowly pull the two hands apart, thus stretching the penis. Hold to the count of ten.
6. Release the grip on the head of the penis and use the hand on the base to whip your penis from side to side against the thigh of each leg. Then, repeat step five and six at least three times.
7. Now, repeat the stretching technique of step five but direct the stretch to go to the left side of your body, followed by the whipping. Repeat this set three times.
8. Then do the same thing but stretching towards the right side of your body, followed by the whipping. Repeat this three times.
9. Once again, grip the base of your penis with one hand. This time, place the thumb and index finger (forming an "okay" sign) next to the other hand at the base of the penis. Hold firmly and slide the one hand only toward the tip of the penis, forcing blood toward the head, causing an engorgement and stretching of the central chamber.
10. Then switch hands and use the other to stretch the penis. Keep alternating until you have repeated the stretch a dozen times.
11. When you are finished, hold the penis at its base with one hand and swing it in circles a dozen times both clockwise and counterclockwise.

II. THE INSIDE (Reproductive System)

Like the female's internal, sexual anatomy, the male's sexual organs are all housed within the pelvic cavity, with the exception of the testicles, located in the externally hanging scrotum. The internal anatomy of a man includes the *prostate* and *testicles*.

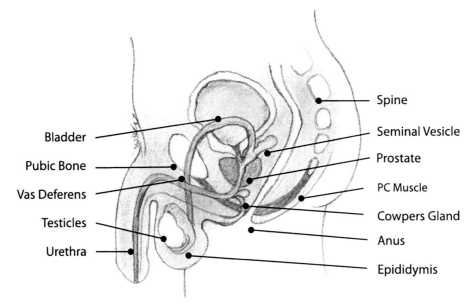

Side view of the male sexual anatomy

THE PROSTATE is the male equivalent of the female G-spot. It's about the size of a chestnut and is attached at its base to the bottom of the bladder. The ejaculatory ducts from each testicle, as well as the urethra, pass through the prostate. The prostate secretes most of the seminal fluid, a thin alkaline substance that neutralizes the acidic environment of the vagina. This fluid combines with the secretions from the seminal vesicles and the sperm from the testicles before flowing into the urethra.

Prior to ejaculation, the penis usually releases a few drops of a clear, mucous-like fluid (secreted from the Cowper's Gland located below the prostate) that exits first–commonly called "pre-cum." This fluid is not semen or sperm.

The prostate can be accessed internally through the anus *or* externally by touching the slight indentation in the perineum, located halfway between the anus and testicles.

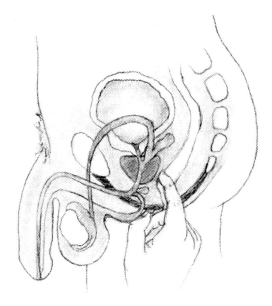

Accessing the prostate

THE TESTICLES are located in the scrotum and have two functions: to produce sperm and secrete sex hormones, or testosterone. Sperm are produced in the seminiferous tubules, highly coiled tubes that form the bulk of the testes. Each testicle is suspended by a spermatic cord that houses muscle fibers, nerves, blood vessels, and the vas deferens. The vas deferens is cut and tied during a *vas*-ectomy to prevent sperm from leaving the testicles.

When a man becomes aroused, his sperm moves from the testicles through the vas deferens tube and into the prostate gland. The vas deferens transfers sperm to the urethra, where secretions from the seminal vesicle and prostate join to form the ejaculate. To protect the sperm from the acidic environment of the urethra, the two Cowper's Glands secrete a clear, alkaline fluid into the urethra. The seminal vesicles also secrete an alkaline fluid that makes up about two-thirds of the seminal fluid. Once combined with this secretion, high in fructose, the sperm are energized and can propel themselves towards their goal of impregnating an egg.

EXERCISE:

Testicle Massage

As with any part of the body, including glands and organs, the best way to assure optimum health of the testicles is through proper nutrients and basic yoga postures. One such position, where the body is bent at the waist with the hands reaching for the floor, creates a massaging of the organs, glands, and muscles in and around the pelvis. Another way to assure testicular health is through direct massage, which increases the production of testosterone, sperm, and seminal fluids.

1. Rub your hands together to warm them.

2. Stretch the skin of the scrotum in various directions.

3. Place the fingertips of both hands beneath your testicles with your thumbs on top. Now massage one testicle in each hand by rolling them between your fingertips and thumbs.

4. With your thumb and forefinger, make a ring around the scrotum just above the testicles. This position tends to squeeze the testicles tightly together. Then gently pull and stretch the testicles towards the floor.

5. Use your other hand to apply a light-pressured massage to one testicle at a time, massaging in small circular motions.

6. Continue this exercise for three to five minutes, two or three times per week. If there is excessive discomfort, ease the amount of pressure on the pull or the massage. If excessive discomfort persists, cease the exercise altogether and consult your physician.

FEMALE AND MALE

Although men and women have sexual anatomy appearing unique to their gender, they also share some of the same anatomical features. Some similarities include the *urethra* (which empties the bladder from the body), the *perineum* (the group of muscles at the base of the torso), the *PC muscle* (the primary muscle of the *perineum* region), the *ring muscles* (the muscles that form a ring around orifices such as the anus), and the *nipples* (which are excitation points for the chest, breast, and heart chakra–as well as the genitals).

THE URETHRA in both the males and females is the long, slender tube that runs from the bladder to the exit point of the genitals where urination takes place. In the male, the urethra runs through the center of the penis and exits at the tip, while in the female, it exits at the small node just below the clitoris.

Infections of the urethra or bladder are not uncommon amongst women, especially if there is a history of sexual trauma. It's also common to get such infections from not using adequate amounts of lubrication or from excessive friction from making love for prolonged periods. Infections are also caused when making love to a new partner, wherein your body has not yet adapted to the organisms within your partner's body.

THE PERINEUM is the group of muscles, including the PC-muscle, in men and women located in the region between the genitals and the anus. When properly stimulated, this area can generate a great deal of pleasure, as it possesses a large number of nerve endings. When stroking this area for a lengthy duration, it's best to use a lubricant.

A man's prostate gland can be indirectly stimulated by pressing straight into the perineum and towards the man's navel. In a woman, the muscles of the perineum also play an important role in sexual arousal and orgasm, since some of the muscles of this region extend to and envelop parts of the clitoris. In fact, a woman's orgasm is triggered in part by her perineum muscles vibrating on the clitoris and vestibular bulbs.

THE PC (pubo-coccygeus) MUSCLE is part of the perineum and may be the most important single muscle for healthy sexuality. It is also the muscle contracted and relaxed during "Kegel" exercises. Unfortunately, most people, including women, don't know where it's located, let alone, what it does. The PC muscle can enhance sexual wellness in numerous ways. It can be used to enlarge the male penis, tone the female vaginal canal, prevent energy leaks from the sexual organs and anus, massage the prostate, and prevent ejaculation.

When tightening and relaxing a well-toned PC muscle, a male can make the penis jump slightly without use of the hand. For a female, the tightening and relaxing of a well-toned PC muscle is experienced as the contraction of the vaginal walls. In fact, some women can fully arouse the penis and bring a man to orgasm during intercourse without any pelvic movement, just by the unique, rhythmic contractions of a well-toned PC muscle.

The PC muscle is located between the genitals and the anus. It extends from the base of the spine (where it connects to the tailbone) to the front of the body (where it connects to the pubic bone). The PC muscle controls the opening and closing of the urethra, the seminal canal, the vagina, and the anus. It also increases blood flow to the genitals. Proper use of this muscle can increase early stages of arousal and the intensity of an orgasm, as well as the effectiveness of energy movement.

> *"The woman should ever strive to close and constrict the yoni until it holds the lingam as with a finger, opening and shutting at her pleasure, and finally, acting as the hand of the Gopi girl who milks the cow."*
>
> *–Ananga Ranga*

EXERCISE:

PC Muscle or Kegel Exercise

Contracting the PC muscle is arguably the most important exercise to enhance sexual health. This one, simple exercise tones the vaginal walls, tightens the ring muscle around the mouth of the vagina, and enhances control of the muscle most instrumental in creating an in-jaculation. Tightening of the PC muscle sends a surge of energy up the spine just moments before an ejaculation. The more toned this muscle, the more effective the energy pumping during an in-jaculation.

1. Sit comfortably and do some slow, deep breathing. Completely relax your belly, abdomen, and perineum regions.

2. Concentrate on the muscles in the perineum region, and gently contract the PC muscle. You should be able to feel your anus contracting, as well as a slight pulling sensation in the genitals.

3. Hold your contraction for five seconds, and then release for five seconds. Repeat this exercise ten times with light contractions and then ten more with full contractions.

4. These contractions might cause a tingling sensation up your spine or some quivering in the perineum region.

5. Eventually concentrate on the difference between using the PC muscle to pull on the tailbone versus using it to pull on the genitals. Then practice alternating between pulling the tailbone and the genitals. Then practice pulling both areas simultaneously.

THE RING MUSCLES are the round sphincter muscles located around the openings of major organ systems, including the eyes, mouth, anus, perineum, and genitals. It is clear, even to the western medical world, that the body's ring muscles are important to a person's overall health. This concept is not new to Taoists, who were well versed in the importance and power of the ring muscles. Taoist master, Mantak Chia states, *"For the body to be in optimal health, it is very important that all the ring muscles contract simultaneously, establishing the inner rhythm and structure of the body. This synchronized movement pumps energy throughout the body."*

The sphincter muscle encircles the anus and the vagina on a woman and the anus and base of the penis on a man. When the pelvic muscles are tensed, as during orgasm, they contract and pull up the sphincter muscles, which is the body's way of preparing to release an orgasm. To reverse the tensing, try deliberately pushing *down* and *out* on the muscle for a few seconds (as though you were urinating) and then relax the muscle. While you are doing the pushing, be sure to breathe deeply and calmly. Practice this "push and relax" exercise, a few times during intercourse. Again, this tends to reverse the effects of pelvic tensing.

Anyone interested in maintaining good health and particularly students of sacred sexuality should exercise their ring muscles to assure their tone. The entire process takes only a few minutes and can usually be done anywhere at any time. Again, there are several ring muscles in the body, so exercise one at a time by moving downward from head to tailbone.

The Eyes: Practice rapidly blinking the eyes by squeezing them shut firmly and then opening them wide. This is believed to improve vision and the health of the eyes, as well as create greater alertness by stimulating the nerves. Practice this exercise for about thirty seconds.

The Mouth: Contract the mouth by sucking the cheeks into the mouth and hold. Then relax the mouth and repeat at least one to two dozen times.

The Perineum and Genitals: Simultaneously contract the perineum and sexual organs (vagina or penis and testicles). Contract and release the muscles in the region of the perineum and observe how the genitals will contract as well. In fact, if you are sensitive and are doing the exercise properly, you will also feel the tailbone contracting towards the genitals. This contraction occurs because the PC muscle connects the pubic and coccyx bones at the perineum. Strengthening the muscles in this region helps in the prevention of energy-leakage through the genitals or anus. Furthermore, as these muscles develop, they become a useful pump for moving sexual energy upwards through the body.

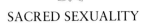

The Anus: Practice contracting the anus, which should be done without too much assistance from the gluteus maximus (butt) muscles. Contract the anus and then relax. Do this at least one to two dozen times.

All Ring Muscles Together: Lastly, it's crucial to synchronize and work all of the ring muscles at the same time. So practice contracting and relaxing all of them simultaneously. It may take time to develop the ability to be aware of their simultaneous contraction. Nevertheless, contract and relax them all together at least one to two dozen times. This exercise will strengthen the body and send surges of energy through the nervous system and energy systems.

THE CHEST, BREASTS AND NIPPLES are an essential part of any discussion of the human sexual anatomy. These points of excitation are such a vital part of sexuality that some women can be brought to orgasm just by stimulation of their nipples. At the very least, stimulation of the nipples will evoke a genital response in most people, especially women. The best way to a woman's yoni (vagina) is through her heart (breasts). And to touch her heart is to open her soul. The woman's yoni will then begin to vibrate in response to the quickening in her heart and breasts.

The intense level of sensitivity some individuals have in their nipples results in part from an energetic connection between the ears, nipples, ovaries, and vaginal walls. Stimulation of one, therefore, can lead to a heightened level of arousal in the others.

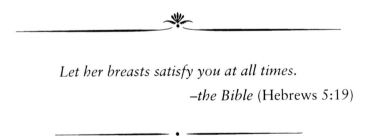

Let her breasts satisfy you at all times.

–the Bible (Hebrews 5:19)

When the breasts and nipples are stimulated, it sends a surge of energy to the heart center (chakra). The breasts and nipples act as sensors for the heart center: carefully checking out the environment, looking for any signals to send to the heart, and letting it know when it's safe to open or when it should shut down. Therefore, these heart sensors should be treated with the utmost love and care.

The breasts and nipples not only *send* signals to the heart center but they also *receive* signals from the heart. When the heart feels authentic love, the breasts and nipples respond more fully. If treated properly, it is not uncommon for a person's nipples to become pleasurably responsive–even if they had not been so in the past. If you want someone else to know how you like to have your breasts and/or nipples touched, first explore them yourself. When washing, be conscious of your breast and nipples. Stroke them with love and perhaps even sensuality. Occasionally give your breasts a massage with an inward and upward motion, lifting and toning them. Avoid treating the nipples roughly during massage or sexual contact because over time the pain programs them to shut down. Excessive sucking on the nipples can also have a numbing effect, which occurs in some women after prolonged breast-feeding. On the other hand, once a *deeper* state of sexual arousal is well under way, a firmer touch might feel right.

EXERCISE:
Healing Breast Massage

Again, women should take the time to get in touch with their breasts: massaging, exploring, healing, loving, and stimulating them–beyond the usual self-applied breast exam. A woman should regularly feel her breasts and/or practice healing breast exercises to maintain healthy breasts.

This exercise, known by Taoists as the "Deer Exercise," elevates a woman's overall health and vitality. But it should *never* be done by a pregnant woman. By practicing it, a woman can ease her menstrual discomforts, tone her breasts, and heal or energize her ovaries. This exercise, which is best done in the morning, is also beneficial for a low libido because it stimulates the entire endocrine system. When performed daily, this breast massage can balance the hormones and regulate the menstrual cycle. Taoists call it "turning back the blood" because, as with nursing, the breast activity in this exercise helps prevent menstruation. As a form of breast massage, the Deer Exercise is also said to prevent cysts, tumors, and breast cancer.

1. Sit comfortably in a chair with the heel of one foot pressed up against the opening of the vagina. The heel should apply steady, firm pressure on the clitoris. If your leg will not bend far enough, then use a tennis ball (or something similar).
2. Rub your hands together to warm them and activate their healing energy.
3. Place your palms on your breasts to feel the heat.
4. Rub your breasts around the outer portion of the nipples in a circular

motion (avoiding direct contact on the nipples). Massage thirty-six times in an upward and outward direction.

5. While doing the breast rotations, add contractions of your PC muscle. As you hold the contraction and rub the breasts, count to six. Then, relax the contraction for a count of six but keep on rubbing. Repeat the contracting and relaxing three dozen times. This will assist in creating an association between your breasts and reproductive organs and glands.

6. After consistent practice of this exercise, you should notice a difference in your menstrual flow. The flow might even cease. If you stop doing the exercises regularly, the menstrual flow will probably return.

Does Size Really Matter?

The image of oversized female breasts or male genitals dates back to a time when sexual anatomy was first used to symbolize fertility. Voluptuous goddesses and gods with large phalluses were believed to once roam the earth. Humans with such endowments were believed to be descendents of these divine beings.

In the context of sacred sexuality, however, the size and shape of a person's body or its parts, such as breast and penis, make no difference because the focus is on the soul. **Even with only a little understanding of sacred sex, most people would not prioritize quantity (size) over quality.**

Time and again studies have proven that race or height only generally determines breast or genital size. This means that despite social beliefs and media hype, the sizes of people's sexual organs are not determined by, nor reflected in, the sizes of their noses, feet, hands, or bodies. One of the more recent studies of men with extra large feet discovered that these men still have average erections of five to six inches. Surveys to determine if race has a bearing on the size of genitals only proved that men of *all* races remain within the same average, varying only by as much as one inch.

From the standpoint of sacred sexuality, there are two crucial points concerning genital size. First, the genitals should be as compatible in size as possible because there are more healing benefits to intercourse when the genitals of a man and woman fit well. Compatibility of genital size allows more skin-to-skin contact and permits the partners to relax more fully, knowing that neither one has to be intimidated by oversize or has to do extra work to compensate for undersize. Second, the sexual experience is enhanced when partners find each other's bodies, including the genitals, to be visually appealing.

Ejaculation

Female ejaculations, according to medical science, are still a doubtful occurrence. In fact, many medical experts are not certain that a woman even has an orgasm, let alone an ejaculation. They especially deny that a woman can release an ejaculate fluid. Yet, this fact was not unknown to the ancients. In classic writings on sacred sexuality, a woman's ejaculate fluid is called *amrita*, or "divine nectar."

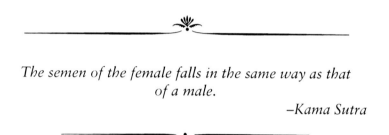

The semen of the female falls in the same way as that of a male.

–*Kama Sutra*

Despite the denial of many medical experts, a modern laboratory analysis found that a woman does indeed release an ejaculate from the vestibular (Bartholin) glands (located towards the lower portion of the vaginal opening) and the paraurethral (Skene's) glands (located towards the upper portion of the vaginal opening). The analysis confirmed that the ejaculate was unique and contained neither urine nor vaginal secretions. However, it was found to be high in prostatic acid, phosphatase, and gluconal–similar to a male's ejaculate. Still, this release of ejaculate fluid by a woman is relatively rare. When it occurs, it's usually from the extended stimulation of the G-spot. In other words, the amrita is an alchemical by-product created in the sexual fires within the female body and triggered by proper stimulation of the G-spot.

A woman's ejaculate, or nectar, varies in color from clear to slightly opaque and varies in taste from astringent to sweet or has no taste at all. A woman often inhibits ejaculation because of the sensation of urination when she is about to release the amrita. So she consciously or unconsciously tenses up and holds back. But when a woman lets go, she can actually have an ejaculation. The quantity of fluid can range from a teaspoon to a cupful.

The amount partly depends on whether her orgasm also triggers a release of her bladder, in which case a larger quantity of fluid is released.

The essential tools to achieve a female ejaculation are as follows:

1. An open and ready mind
2. Total relaxation
3. A well developed PC muscle
4. Patience and persistence

When you are ready to ejaculate, be sure that you are in a comfortable position and that you "push out" on the PC muscles as if urinating. Also, timing is of the essence. You must push out the ejaculate just prior to the peak of your orgasm – not too early and not too late.

If you are already a woman who ejaculates (or soon become one) be sure to inform your partner. Otherwise, being fairly rare among women, it can shock, surprise, or even scare your partner when you ejaculate unexpectedly.

Ancient Taoist masters speak of three waters (or types of fluid) involved in female orgasms. The first water is the lubrication experienced during arousal. The second water is the fluid emitted during normal orgasm. The third water is the female ejaculate released from the sacred spot. All three fluids are a manifestation of shakti energy (divine, female sexual energy), which either the male or female can absorb during lovemaking. Absorption of this energy is one of the most magical aspects of sacred sexuality. Both partners can benefit from absorbing this shakti, or nectar, that revitalizes and nurtures–physically and energetically. For the male, the absorption of shakti energy occurs while he (erect or not) is inside of the female. Absorption of this energy recharges the male even if he has already allowed an orgasm with ejaculation, in which case, he would make sure his lingam remains in her yoni as long as possible after ejaculation. While inserted, he envisions "sipping" the love juices by drawing in his PC muscle and imagining he is breathing in, or absorbing, her essence. Since this is primarily an energetic experience, this absorption process is reduced by the use of a condom but not completely eliminated.

The basic steps for ejaculating are as follows:

1. Make sure you feel physically and mentally prepared.
2. Stimulate the G-spot enough to engorge with fluid.
3. Keep some pressure on the G-spot while you stimulate the clitoris to point of orgasm.
4. Then, as you reach a high clitoral orgasm, release the pressure on the G-spot and push.

Male ejaculations actually occur in two stages. The first stage is the ejaculation preparation stage, wherein the seminal fluid, including the sperm, flows into the urethral bulb. The prostate enlarges, as it fills with secretions, until it is full and cannot contain any more tension. The prostate, seminal vesicles, vas deferens, and the two urethral sphincters (internal and external) experience a series of contractions, which keep the seminal fluid in the urethral bulb. These strong rhythmic contractions also occur in the muscles surrounding the bulb and the root of the penis and continue along the entire urethral passage. This process gives a man the sensation that signals ejaculation is imminent.

The second stage is the actual release of fluid, wherein semen (trapped in the urethral bulb) is released as the external urethral sphincter relaxes. The sperm and other fluids then pass through the urethra and out of the penis, after which the prostate shrinks back to its normal size. Once ejaculation is over (which takes about five to ten seconds) and engorgement eases, the internal sphincter relaxes and urine can once again enter the urethra. The average amount of sperm released by a male is about one teaspoonful.

The amount of fluid ejaculated can be increased. The most common methods are as follows:

1. Refrain from ejaculating every time you have sex or are aroused. Instead, ejaculate only once in every three arousals.
2. Dissolve a slice of fresh ginseng in your mouth once per day (after consulting a naturopath or medical doctor).
3. Massage the testicles regularly.
4. Drink plenty of water on a consistent basis.

The flavor of semen can vary from person to person, but it can be enhanced by the eating of fresh cinnamon, pineapple or licorice root on a regular basis. Cigarettes and alcohol should be avoided. Diet also has an effect on the taste of semen. Meats tend to make semen saltier; dairy products add a bitter taste, and a vegetarian diet sweetens the taste of semen.

During the second stage of ejaculation, the first fluid released from the penis (commonly referred to as "pre-cum") is a secretion from the Cowper's glands, which are two pea-sized glands located between the shaft of the penis and the prostate gland. The fluid released from the Cowper's glands alkalizes the acidic environment of the urethra for the benefit of the sperm that will soon travel through.

The sperm are then released from the testicles, where they are mixed with semen from the seminal vesicle and the prostate gland. These two fluids combined are released during ejaculation.

If the PC muscle is strong, it can (during the contractions) put enough pressure on the channel that passes the prostate gland to prevent semen from passing through. The body can recycle the preserved seminal fluid and transport these juices (filled with nutrients and life-force) into the bloodstream via the lymphatic duct. Semen retention, of course, nourishes the body because instead of expelling this energy, it is reabsorbed into the system. This technique of using of the PC muscle to prevent the passing of semen is crucial to turning an e-jaculation into an in-jaculation.

Practicing in-jaculation, or "ejaculation control," is one of the best methods for preventing premature ejaculation or premature orgasms even without an ejaculation. Premature ejaculation can be defined as "having an ejaculation or orgasm before preferred." Premature ejaculation can be caused by emotional issues and by such physical issues as excessive tensing of the muscles within the pelvic region. Although this problem is thought to be a concern exclusively for men, women too can reach orgasms before they prefer. Almost all men and women have experienced premature ejaculation at least once in their lives. The primary concern, however, is that when a man experiences a premature ejaculation, it usually means he cannot remain erect, which for some couples is perceived as inhibiting their ability to continue their sexual encounter. In such cases, a man's premature ejaculation is as frustrating to women as it is to men.

Taoists believe that semen (*ching*) is a man's most valuable life-force energy; that semen generates life; and that by reversing the process of expelling semen, a man can regenerate his health and vitality. Likewise, excessive semen loss can damage the nervous system, weaken muscles, harm digestion, deplete the body's vitality, and cause premature aging. After all, an average ejaculation contains 50-250 million sperm cells. If each one were to fertilize an egg, it would only take a few ejaculations to populate a large country. This common energy loss is why orgasms are referred to as "*le petit morte*," meaning "the little death." Therefore, Taoists clearly discourage unnecessary loss of semen through excessive ejaculations. The Taoist formula for how often a healthy male should allow ejaculation is as follows: *healthy* males in their teens can ejaculate twice per day; at age thirty, once per day; at forty, once every few days; at fifty, once every five days; at sixty, once every ten days; and, at seventy, once per month. The number of days in between ejaculations should be doubled for *unhealthy* males.

In sexual intercourse, semen must be regarded as a most precious substance. By saving it, a man protects his very life. Whenever he does ejaculate, the loss of semen must then be compensated by absorbing the woman essence.

–Peng-Tze *(Secrets of the Jade Bedroom)*

Remember, ejaculations and orgasms are not the same. An ejaculation is purely physiological, an involuntary muscle spasm. An orgasm, on the other hand, can be a spiritual, energetic, and physiological experience. In fact, ejaculations and orgasms can be separated at the moment of climactic arousal. This separation process allows the male to experience multiple ejaculations without orgasms or, better yet, multiple orgasms without ejaculation, which prevents the loss of the male's vital fluids, energy, and erection.

When attempting to separate ejaculations from orgasms, the key is to remain relaxed despite the tension of arousal. The male also needs to visualize relaxing the soft tissue and muscles within the penis, as well as spreading the hot sexual energy (with hands and mind) from the genitals throughout the body. Finally, it's essential to keep building sexual arousal using techniques for delaying ejaculation until the body spontaneously experiences a non-ejaculatory orgasm.

EXERCISES:

Delaying Ejaculation

Delaying an *ejaculation* is *not*, by definition, the same as having an *in-jaculation*. But there are several techniques for delaying a male ejaculation that *can assist* in creating an in-jaculation. These include breath control, pumping the prostate, pulling on the testicles, pinching the head of the penis, and muscle relaxation. Some of these techniques are more effective than others. It should be remembered, however, that the use of techniques that literally *block* the release of fluids (such as manually pinching the head of the penis) can result in various discomforts or temporary swelling of the testicles.

1. BREATH CONTROL

When most men approach the point of orgasm, they breathe heavier and faster, while tending to hold their breath to some degree when they actually cum. One way to "trick" the body into releasing the urge to orgasm is to change the breathing pattern to slow, deep, and rhythmical. This pattern reverses the flow of sexual energy by sending a signal to the brain that there is less excitation than is actually present.

2. PUMPING THE PROSTATE

When a man becomes sexually stimulated, the prostate engorges with sexual fluids until these fluids are released upon ejaculation, at which point the prostate propels the fluids out of the body. Pump the prostate by squeezing and releasing the PC muscle while taking in long, deep breaths with each contraction. It's important to squeeze at the first urge to ejaculate. One long squeeze might be enough, but get into the habit of doing a few to be certain the energy has moved out of the genitals. While pumping the prostate or practicing any other form of ejaculation prevention, cease all movement and stimulation until the urge to ejaculate has passed. The prostate can also be pumped manually by pressing in the perineum. Applying deep pressure to the perineum area by hand exerts pressure on the prostate, alleviating the urge to ejaculate.

3. PULLING ON THE TESTICLES

Most men can experience some pulling on the scrotum without any discomfort. This practice involves pulling the entire scrotum (testicle sac) downward, toward the feet–gently but firmly for about fifteen seconds. When a man is about to have an ejaculation, the testicles are drawn up into his body. Pulling them downward sends a message to the brain that the urge to ejaculate has passed. Therefore, pulling down on the scrotum reverses the process of ejaculation. As with the use of the PC muscle, timing is everything, so this technique must be used *before* "the point of no return."

4. PINCHING THE HEAD OF THE PENIS

If you choose to practice this technique while having intercourse, withdraw the penis just before the "point of no return." Then, hold the head of the penis firmly until some of the arousal subsides. To hold the head of the penis properly, the tip should be against the palm with the heel of the hand on the backside of the penis and the fingertips clamped onto the frenulum or underside–just below the head.

5. MUSCLE RELAXATION

This technique involves becoming very aware of what's going on in your body during sexual stimulation–especially in your muscles and breathing as you approach an orgasm. Are you holding your breath? Are you tensing certain muscles and, if so, which ones? If you notice any tension in your mind, breath or body, mentally direct the tensed area to relax. Physically shake your body periodically to dislodge any stuck tension.

Physical Orgasms

The most common type of orgasm is the physical, peak, orgasm, which usually results from direct stimulation of the penis or clitoris (the female's version of a penis). The physical orgasm results in an ejaculation of fluids and strong sensations within the muscles and nervous system, as well as a brief burst of energy in the pelvis. During this level of orgasm, there are similarities and differences between the physiological responses of a man and woman. The most general similarity is that for both men and women a physical orgasm is basically just an ejaculation. This means that both men and women experience an engorgement of blood to the genital region and a contracting of their muscles and internal organs, not dissimilar to preparing to sneeze–which is why a physical orgasm is sometimes referred to as a "pelvic sneeze." The man's testicles contract, as do the woman's clitoris and vaginal canal. The orgasmic buildup culminates as several quick, spasm-like contractions, followed by a release of energy and fluids. This "climax" of energy buildup and explosion is what most people experience as an orgasm.

There are two general stages (build-up and release) of a physical orgasm. These are activated by two different parts of the nervous system. The arousal and stimulation are connected to the parasympathetic portion of the autonomic nervous system. The muscular contractions and orgasmic release are connected to the sympathetic portion of the autonomic nervous system.

More specifically, there are actually four stages of a physical orgasm: arousal, plateau, release, and resolution. During arousal, the genitals and surrounding tissue become engorged with blood, and the woman's vaginal canal becomes moist with droplets of fluid. During the plateau, the clitoris

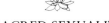
and penis become more fully erect, and the man may release a few drops of pre-cum (from the Cowper's gland). The woman's uterus lifts away from the pelvic floor, and the upper part of her vaginal canal balloons out. During the actual release, there are numerous muscular contractions in the local muscles and an internal releasing of the trapped, engorged blood that now spreads back into the body; then there is a release of fluids from the penis or vagina. Finally, when the stage of resolution is reached, the muscles and organs return to their relaxed state, heavy breathing subsides, and the penis and clitoris become flaccid.

In addition to the physiological responses, there are deeper and more varied dimensions to physical stimulation and orgasm than most people are aware of. Although the clitoris and penis are the most commonly used keys to orgasm, orgasms can also be reached through the stimulation of other portions of the genitals, such as a woman's G-spot and a man's prostate. The same holds true for the various parts of the woman's yoni. A woman can have an orgasm by stimulation of her cervix, which is often triggered by insertion of the penis deeply enough to rub against the cervix. In fact, any part of the human body can reach an orgasm–as long as the recipient is receptive and there is proper stimulation.

Even though men and women have orgasmic similarities, there are differences as well. Two such differences are the length of time it takes to build up to an orgasm and the duration of the orgasm. In both cases, the woman's process is considerably longer. One reason for this additional time arises from the woman's different pelvic structure and longer pelvic muscles. It takes more time to engorge the woman's pelvic area with blood than it does a man's.

Another difference between the male and female orgasm is the short-lived, intense peak of the male orgasm, biologically necessary to force semen deep into the vaginal canal. Women, on the other hand, have several levels and types of physical orgasms.

Building an Orgasm

To build an intense orgasm for your partner (or yourself), bring your partner as close as possible to orgasm and keep him (or her) on that plateau, not allowing an actual release. You can prevent your partner from "going over the top" by changing rhythm, pace or pressure. Once your partner comes down a little, repeat the process. Then draw your partner up again, getting him (or her) as close as possible to peaking without going over the top. Assist your partner in riding the plateau just before orgasm. Repeat this practice at least three times or perhaps more. Each time the energy is built up, it increases the amount of physical, emotional, and spiritual energy to be released. The intent is to build a constant increase in excitement to intensify the resulting orgasm.

The secret to building an orgasm without going past the point of no return is to know when your partner is about to climax. The closer you can bring your partner to the point of orgasm (but not release) with the greatest number of repetitions of this process, the more the ecstatic energy builds, resulting in an intense, sustained orgasm.

Once you deepen the level of orgasm, the energy spreads, and the pleasure increases. The whole nervous system is thereby flooded with life-force. There are various means of preventing ejaculation and creating an in-jaculation to deepen the level of orgasm. Some of the most common techniques are as follows:

- Develop self-control and a heightened awareness of sexual feelings and physiological sensations during each moment.
- Reduce stimulation before reaching the point of no return.
- Contract and hold the PC muscle while breathing slowing and deeply.
- Focus on the pull, rather than the push, of the penile thrusts. Also, relax the buttock muscles and slow down breathing.
- Apply firm pressure to the prostate (through the perineum) to help interrupt an ejaculation.
- Squeeze the scrotum gently, pulling it down for about 15-30 seconds.
- Hold the penis at the frenulum–just below the head of the penis (about an inch down from the tip). With one finger bent under and the thumb behind the head of the penis, squeeze the frenulum firmly for fifteen to thirty seconds until the erection subsides.
- Stop all stimulation until the urge to ejaculate subsides.
- Taoists recommend practice of the "sets of nine" penetrations exercise (described in this book).

Exercises for the Body

The practice of sacred sexuality includes having a healthy physical lifestyle. This lifestyle might involve eating lighter meals, abstaining from drugs and alcohol, and doing some form of exercise, such as yoga. Yoga exercises help you to maintain a more vigorous and healthy body and cultivate more energy. Stretching and practicing yoga can help you become aware of and release any, or all, body tensions, thus awakening greater sexual pleasure. Most of the following exercises are equally good for men or women.

EXERCISE:

Pelvic Thrust

There are a few strategic regions of the body where energy is most often blocked. The pelvis is one such region. Yet the freedom of flow to this region is important to the overall health of the body. It has always been a common practice in native cultures to exercise and open the pelvic energy flow, as evident in the classic belly dancer or hula dancer. In western cultures, however, we have restrained our pelvises by tying up our tummies with girdles and overly tightened abdominal muscles. As recently as the 1950's, Elvis Presley shocked America with pelvic movements that, at the time, were perceived as "sexual" behavior. Just a little freedom of movement in the pelvis, and he became a controversy because the pelvis is associated with sexual energy. The following is one of the most effective exercises for freeing up the muscles and energy of the pelvic region. This exercise is fun but blatantly "pelvic" or sexual in appearance.

1. Stand with your feet a little wider than shoulders' distance apart.
2. Slowly move your pelvis in a circular motion to warm up the muscles.
3. Now put your hands out in front of you at naval level, and cock your tailbone back.
4. Then pull your hands towards your hips as you thrust your tailbone forward. This should simulate the sexual thrusting a man does when he is having intercourse with his partner from behind.
5. As you thrust your hips forward, exhale with a "huh" sound.
6. Repeat the thrusting a dozen times. Then on the exhale, replace the "huh" with a resounding "yes" on each thrust. Repeat this at least two dozen times.

EXERCISE:

Yoga: Sun Salutation

The sun salutation is easily the most common set of yoga postures and is used within nearly all styles of yoga. The reason for its popularity lies in the fact that it encompasses an effective and efficient set of postures that relax and stretch nearly every muscle group. The sun salutation is a great warm up or cool down exercise or can be used as an exercise independent of any other workout. It's good for the circulatory and lymphatic systems. The sun salutation is also easy to memorize, since many of the postures are repeated for the opposite side of the body once you reach the halfway point of the exercise.

While practicing the sun salutation, breathe in a manner than works for you. Or you might try inhaling as you move out of each posture and exhaling as you stretch into each posture. Each posture should be held for at least five to ten seconds.

1. Stand straight with your knees unlocked. Hold your hands in a praying position over your heart as you center into a moment of dedication.

2. Stretch your hands above your head, and lean back as far as is comfortable. Tighten your butt to support your low back.

3. Slowly bend forward (at the hip, not the waist) and bring your hands to the floor, even if you have to bend your knees to do so.

4. Keep your hands flat on the floor as you slide your right foot back as far as you can and drop your right knee to the floor. Raise your hands above your head, and arch your upper body back.

5. Straighten your body (into "push-up" position) and then raise your butt to the sky until you form an inverted "V" shape. In this position, bring your heels flat to the ground, let your head hang, and push your chest towards your legs.

6. Bring your hands to the floor in front of you, and slide your left foot back next to your right, keeping your body straight (such as in a "push-up" position). Then lower your knees to the ground, sit back on your ankles, and stretch your chest towards the floor.

7. Slide your chest along the floor until you have stretched your body out again, let your hips set on the ground, and arch your upper body back.

8. Straighten your body again (back into "push-up" position) and then raise your butt to the sky until you form an inverted "V" shape. In this

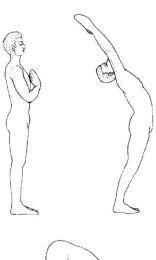
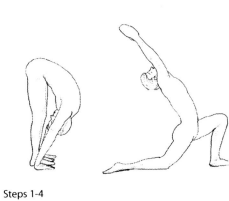

Steps 1-4

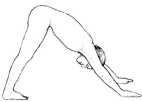
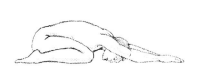

Steps 5-6

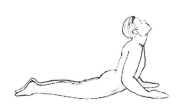
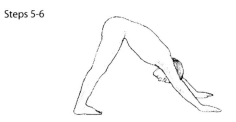

Steps 7-8

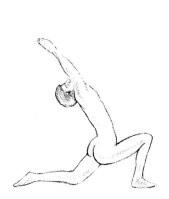

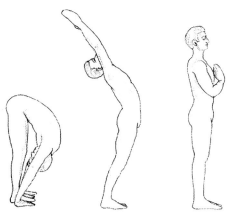

Steps 9-12

position, bring your heels flat to the ground, let your head hang, and push your chest towards your legs.

9. Once again, straighten your body into "push-up" position and then bring your right foot forward and place it between your hands. Drop your left knee to the floor, raise your hands above your head, and arch your upper body back, exactly as you did in step four.

10. Bring your hands to the floor on each side of your right foot, slide your left foot next to your right, and allow your body to hang forward. This is a repeat of the posture in step three.

11. Slowly lift your torso, raise your hands above your head and arch back, exactly as you did in step two.

12. Bring your hands back into praying position in front of your heart and spend a moment in prayerful thanksgiving. This posture returns you to step number one.

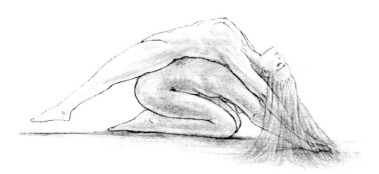

Excercise to open the body

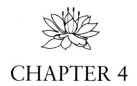

CHAPTER 4

Your Energy Systems

Esoteric Anatomy 101

Since sacred sexuality focuses on the whole person, beyond the physical body, the practitioner should understand the body's basic, esoteric (hidden or invisible) anatomy. The following includes information on the human energy systems, such as meridians (commonly used in acupuncture), chakras (primary energy centers), and kundalini energy (that runs along the spine and activates the nervous system). These systems (along with other portions of the esoteric anatomy not as yet mentioned) are individually and/or collectively referred to as the body's "energy systems."

Information on esoteric anatomy is important for a thorough understanding of the human body. This knowledge is vital during the practice of sacred sexuality, where expansion into higher levels of orgasm and ecstasy involves the esoteric anatomy, even more so than the physical.

Unless you go beyond your biology you will never know your soul.

–Osho

THE MERIDIANS

Traditional Chinese medicine teaches that there are twelve major organ meridians in the human body. These meridians are like veins of energy that run through the head, torso, and limbs. There are also another eight meridians, referred to as "extraordinary" veins or channels. Each of the twelve (plus eight) meridians is fed by the body's major chakras, which are like energy power plants.

All of the meridians can become electrified and awakened with ecstatic, orgasmic energy. Even so, when experiencing an orgasm, it would be nearly impossible to tell the difference between electrified meridians versus an activated nervous system, as both systems can become charged, resulting in tingling sensations and warm rushes of energy.

EXERCISE:

Energy Shake

There are several ways to activate the energy systems of the body. One of the easiest methods has always been used by native cultures around the world. Activating the energy systems is effective for loosening muscle tensions, opening blocked chi (energy) in the body, and creating greater blood flow to the organs and glands.

1. Remove all of your clothing.
2. Play rhythmic music, preferably music that builds in pace.
3. Slowly stretch the muscles in your neck and torso until they are warmed and loosened.
4. Slowly loosen your muscles by gently shaking your legs and arms. Then allow every part of your body to move. Especially allow your breast (women) and genitals (men) to bounce freely.
5. Once you feel your body is loosened up, begin shaking more vigorously. Shake your fingers, hands, and arms, as well as you feet and legs.
6. Shake your body wildly for at least five minutes.
7. When you are done, sit or lie still and allow the buzz of energy to permeate your body from head to toe and limb to limb.

THE CHAKRAS AND NADIS

There are seven major chakras, or energy centers, in the body. Counting upward, the first is located at the base of the spine; the second is just below the navel; the third is located at the solar plexus; the fourth (the heart chakra) is located in the center of the chest; the fifth is in the neck; the sixth (commonly called the third eye) is in the lower portion of the forehead; and the seventh (the crown chakra) is at the top of the head.

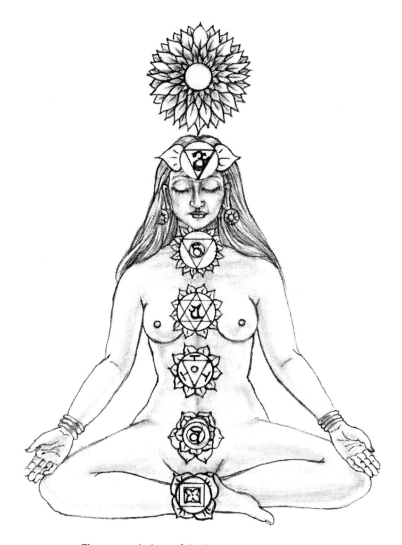

The seven chakras of the human energy systems

During an in-jaculation, a current of energy is sent out from the reproductive organs to the base of the spine. It then travels up the spine to the top of the head–activating most, or all, of the chakras along the way. Once this activation process occurs, each chakra channels energy into the acupuncture meridians and central nervous system. This channeling of energy throughout the body's energy systems and nervous system results in more intense sensations and a full-body experience because orgasmic energy is now transported to every part of the body.

The seven chakras are connected to the central nervous system and spine via small energy channels called "nadis" in Sanskrit. The *nadis* form a web of 72,000 circuits that carry energy throughout the etheric and physical bodies, bridging the two through the central nervous system. The three primary *nadi* channels are called *ida, pingala,* and *sushumna. Ida* and *pingala* represent the feminine (lunar) and masculine (solar) polarities that flow up each side of the spine from the tailbone to the center of the head (forming the caduceus) and then into the left (*ida*) and right (*pingala*) nostrils. *Sushumna* is a *nadi*, or channel, that goes through the central, hollow portion of the spinal column from tailbone to crown of head and assists the movement of cerebral spinal fluid from the spinal sacrum to the inner portion of the cranial bones of the skull. *Sushumna* represents the "Christ Channel" that symbolizes the awakening of the Divine Self, an energetic process commonly referred to as "kundalini rising." This rising is usually experienced as a subtle, ongoing process that occurs in gradual stages or occasionally as a more dramatic spiritual awakening.

Ida can be activated by breathing through the left nostril, which evokes a calm, compassionate energy. *Pingala* can be stimulated by breathing through the right nostril, which promotes clarity and direction. *Sushumna* can be stimulated into activity by the purification and balanced awakening of *ida* and *pingala* through the alternate breathing of the left and right nostrils–commonly referred to as *pranayama breathing.*

Alternate breathing of each nostril and the activation of *ida* and *pingala* charge the cerebral spinal fluid with positive and negative energy and balance the right and left hemispheres of the brain. As this charged energy rises up the spine, it activates each chakra along the way, which in turn, awakens the correlative endocrine glands and organs. This process also activates the central nervous system and awakens brain cells, resulting in waves of energy and a state of ecstasy. As the chakras are activated, the old unhealed patterns they hold are released and brought to the surface for healing. For this reason, it is vital that the activation of the chakras be done in conjunction with a spiritual practice and *not* merely as a form of energy-activation.

KUNDALINI

Kundalini (coiled serpent) is a manifestation of the life-force that lies mostly dormant at the base of the spine. Usually the body accesses only a minimal amount of its kundalini power–just enough to stay alive. Yet, there remains an entire storehouse of this energy awaiting the moment when it can bring each cell of the body fully to life. An individual can learn to awaken the kundalini and raise it from the sexual, root center to all the other centers, or chakras, of the body. Some call this practice of awakening the kundalini *White Tantra* or *kundalini-shakti.*

The kundalini represents the human soul and the goddess (Shakti) within that yearns to move upward along the spine and meet with the god (Shiva) of the crown center. This reunion creates an ecstatic energy response known as *samadhi,* a bliss that represents and embodies the union dance of Shiva and Shakti–male and female deities of Tantra.

Although kundalini energy is known by many names and has several functions, in the context of this material, the kundalini is commonly referred to as sexual energy (or shakti). Yet the kundalini energy is a life-force that exists beyond the level of sexual energy. In a male, when the kundalini manifests as sexual energy, it is often ignited and released through ejaculation before it has time to reach its incredible potential. Likewise, in a female, the sexual energy is often snuffed out before it has time to build even a faint glow. But when the sexual (kundalini) energy is properly ignited, magnified, and channeled, it can do wondrous things for an individual's health and vitality, as well as awaken profound spiritual experiences.

While unknown to medical science, many practitioners of Tantra maintain that there is a small gland between the rectum and sacrum called the *kunda* gland, where the primary essence of the kundalini energy resides. Medical science does, however, acknowledge that this region has a sacral nerve plexus. When this region is stimulated, manually or energetically, it activates the kundalini flow. You may have discovered this if you've ever fallen on your butt and felt an energy surge move up through your spine. The kundalini energy can be awakened more gently, however, by rocking the pelvis back and forth, as you contract your PC muscle, causing a pumping sensation of the sacrum against this gland.

As the kundalini begins to move, the chakras come to life. The chakras, meridians, and kundalini energy contain the information about your soul's journey as well as any unresolved emotional issues. Therefore, it's essential to balance the following kundalini exercises with grounding techniques. Grounding prevents a feeling of being overwhelmed by the energetic shifts occurring within your being. Grounding also helps to provide the physical, emotional, psychic and spiritual stability to take processing to a higher level.

Breathing Exercises

Strange as it may seem, the development of proper breathing and advanced techniques in breathing are essential for enhancing sexual experiences. Breathing is essential to living. If we don't breath well, we don't live well.

There is one way of breathing that is shameful and constricted. Then there's another way: a breath of love that takes you all the way to infinity.

–Rumi

Breathing properly is one of the best ways to calm the body and center the mind. It also has a direct affect on the nervous system.

The nervous system is divided into two parts: *the central nervous system*, for voluntary (conscious) movements, and *the autonomic nervous system*, which automatically regulates (subconscious) body functions.

The autonomic nervous system is further divided into two parts–the sympathetic and parasympathetic systems. *The sympathetic system* is responsible for our "fight or flight" responses. Fear and/or shallow breathing keep the sympathetic nervous system in control. *The parasympathetic system,* on the other hand, is related to our states of relaxation. Relaxed, deep breathing into the abdomen activates the parasympathetic nervous system. Switching from the stress response of the sympathetic to the parasympathetic system can be accomplished by practicing proper breathing exercises.

There are numerous breathing techniques to relax the body and enhance the sexual experience, but the most applicable can be divided into the following groups:

1. Deep, slow breathing is the most common breathing technique. It promotes a relaxing and meditative level of consciousness, which means it can calm down the urge to ejaculate or orgasm.

2. Hard, fast breathing has a purifying effect on the nervous system and energy systems. This type of breathing also heats up the entire body and increases arousal. The more intense version of hard and fast breathing is sometimes referred to as the "breath of fire." A simpler version of this intense breathing is simply to pant rapidly from the abdomen with an open mouth. This rapid panting activates the energy systems and helps the body become accustomed to heightened states of arousal and spontaneous release.

EXERCISE:

Deep, Slow Breathing

It is believed that slowing your breaths to eight times per minute activates the pituitary gland, which is the master of all other glands. Slowing your breaths to less than four times per minute activates the pineal gland, which opens you up to Divine Inspiration. Therefore, the simplest correct breathing (slow, deep breaths) has positive effects beyond measure.

The healing and rejuvenating power of proper, conscious breathing can improve the quality of your life. The following slow, deep breathing exercise, for example, assists in centering and calming thoughts and fears.

1. Sit in a chair or lie comfortably on your back. Breathe through your nose for this exercise.
2. Exhale all of the air from your abdomen through your nose.
3. Next, inhale deeply as you visualize air being pulled down into your abdomen, filling your ribs, lungs, chest, and throat.
4. Hold your breath for a moment while keeping your body completely relaxed.
5. Exhale slowly, pushing all the air out from your torso. Then hold your breath for a moment before inhaling again.
6. The inhale and exhale, as well as the pauses in between, should all be the same length–about five seconds. You can increase the count over time.

EXERCISE:

Pranayama Breathing

This exercise is the most well-known advanced form of solo breathing. Pranayama breathing is wonderful for clearing energy trapped within the nervous system, as well as any blockages within the psychic center of the head. This exercise balances the left and right, masculine and feminine, sides of the brain and rejuvenates the energy meridians of the body's energy systems.

1. Sit comfortably with your back straight. Take a couple of deep breaths.

2. Place your right hand on your face, and press your right thumb against your right nostril forcing it closed. Then inhale deeply through the left nostril.

3. Press the middle finger of your right hand against your left nostril forcing it closed, and hold your breath for a few seconds. Make sure your face and mouth remain relaxed.

4. Remove your right thumb from the side of your nose, and exhale your breath through your right nostril.

5. Now inhale through your right nostril. Then close your right nostril with your thumb, and hold your breath for a few seconds.

6. Once again, exhale through your left nostril. Continue this process for twelve complete cycles.

EXERCISE:

Breath of Fire

This exercise is referred to as the "breath of fire" because of its intensity and its ability to assist in awakening the kundalini fire. Its power lies in its ability to warm and activate the energy systems and nervous system. This warming, activating ability is a direct result of the purifying breath and abdominal contractions, particularly in the solar plexus and *hara* center, a few inches below the naval.

1. Begin by sitting comfortably and take a series of slow, deep breaths.

2. After taking at least six to twelve deep breaths, fully inhale through your nose and expand the lungs. Then contract your abdominal muscles upward tightly to push the air out through your mouth. This should create a "huh" sound.

3. Next, relax the abdominal muscles (from the solar plexus to the pubic bone) and allow them to drop. You will find that as you release and relax the abdomen, the lungs simultaneously fill with air.

4. Now repeat the last two steps, but contract (which deflates the lungs) and relax (which inflates the lungs) the abdomen faster and faster. After a little practice, it will begin to feel more natural. Air is now

pulled in, pumped out, and pulled in again–rhythmically. Be sure to allow your arms, legs, chest, shoulders, and neck to remain relaxed.

5. Eventually you will find a pace and rhythm that feels right for you. At that point, let the rhythm take over.

6. After a few minutes, conclude the exercise by returning to slow, deep breathing while simultaneously drawing in a feeling of peace and the Divine Presence.

In-jaculation

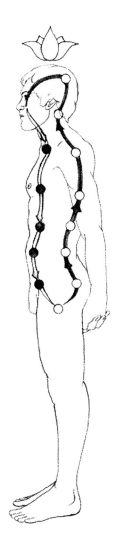

Solo in-jaculation

The most potent force in the universe is creative energy, without which the universe would not exist. The most primal form of creative energy is sexual energy. With this force, we as co-creators can create human beings. Yet, another generative use of this force is available to us as well. We can channel this generative energy from the pelvis up into the skull, a process known as an in-jaculation. The creative force of an in-jaculation feeds life-force to the pineal and pituitary glands, the master controllers of our body. These glands then send messages of cellular renewal to all other glands and organs of the body.

In-jaculation techniques are probably the most important tools for reaching energetic orgasms. They are the first steps for evolving physical orgasms into higher-level (energetic, emotional, mental, and soul-level) orgasms.

Some of the more mainstream teachings on sexuality use the term "in-jaculation" to indicate the process of manually blocking the release of sexual fluids, thus forcing them back into the body before exiting the urethra. This technique might better be referred to as an "ejaculation block" and is not our definition for an in-jaculation. In sacred sexuality, the term in-jaculation refers to a two-step process of separating the orgasm from the ejaculation and drawing the energy from this orgasm inwards and upwards along the spine. Although this process can be practiced by men and women (and is energetically effective for both), it is especially important for males because one of the primary goals is to prevent the loss of semen. The first step in this process is to prevent an ejaculation by simply pausing all stimulation just prior to ejaculation (which means there is little or no semen expelled). In the second step, the buildup of stimulation and excitation in the pelvis and root chakra is then drawn upward from the pelvis and redirected into the higher centers of the body by the use of the mind and specific muscles, such as the PC muscle. If pausing stimulation is not enough to prevent ejaculation, you can also add any of the "ejaculation delay" techniques previously mentioned in Chapter 3.

A crucial factor to the successful practicing of in-jaculation is a thorough knowledge of your body (and that of your partner) so that you heed the signs of an impending orgasm before it's too late. For example, when reaching the point of orgasm, many people hold their breath and tighten their muscles, especially those within the pelvis. This tensing before orgasmic release can be remedied by slow, deep, relaxing breathing. Slowing the breath, alters the faster orgasmic breathing pattern and changes the signals of excitement sent to the brain, while also shifting focus away from sensations of arousal.

The more often in-jaculation is practiced, the safer it is to experience e-jaculations. In-jaculation allows the body to develop a storehouse of energy within the navel center. This energy is accessible by the sexual organs when they are again aroused into activity. An in-jaculation creates pleasurable sensations that differ from an e-jaculation. Besides the usual pelvic pleasuring, there are also subtle sensations that move along the spine and throughout the nervous system. But these sensations are usually noticeable only with continued practice.

Although many forms of sacred sexuality involve controlling the ejaculation, there are also opportune moments when it's best to avoid all forms of resistance, tension, or control and allow the natural process of orgasm to take place. All the tensing that accompanies an in-jaculation should be stopped, and the ejaculation should be unleashed to trigger greater surges of orgasmic energy through the body. A Tantric master never permits a student to hold back from ejaculation for long durations. There is a point when it's better to release all attempts to maintain control and move into a state of complete vulnerability and surrender to whatever is occurring in the moment.

Although giving in to an ejaculation does not mean failure, in Tantra, the masters often prefer to encourage their students to become keenly aware of the ejaculatory process and their own thresholds. Sometimes, the masters teach their students to utilize pressure points to short-circuit ejaculation. Such techniques are used to teach the students how to approach orgasm without tensing. **After practicing total relaxation and ejaculatory control often enough, these techniques allow the students to experience higher levels of orgasm, such as a rapid succession of orgasms without ejaculating.**

EXERCISE:

Basic In-jaculation

The following is a basic exercise for preventing ejaculation by pressing the perineum region and by pausing before an orgasm or ejaculation through the use of self-discipline. This exercise also teaches how to use the PC muscle to pump orgasmic energy up through the body, rather than losing energy through an orgasm or ejaculation.

1. Choose some form of self-stimulation and pleasure yourself until fully aroused.
2. After building sexual stimulation to the point just prior to orgasm or ejaculation, pause all activity.
3. Tighten the PC muscle (or press on the perineum) as you pump the genital energy up the spine. If you press on the perineum, remember that the location and amount of pressure is crucial. If you press too close to the anus, you will not prevent the ejaculation. If you press too close to the scrotum, the semen will enter the bladder and be expelled with urine. The amount of pressure should not be too heavy or too light. The exact location and perfect amount of pressure is best discovered through practice.
4. Next, as you inhale, draw the energy up the back of the body (along the spine) and to the top of the head.
5. As you exhale, allow the energy to flow down the front of the body until it reaches its resting place just below the navel.

6. Repeat this energy circulation at least three times before continuing to stimulate. Then, once an orgasm again draws near, repeat the in-jaculation exercise.

7. You may, or may not, feel sensations moving through your body the first time you practice this exercise. However, feeling sensations in the body is not a prerequisite to moving on to other exercises.

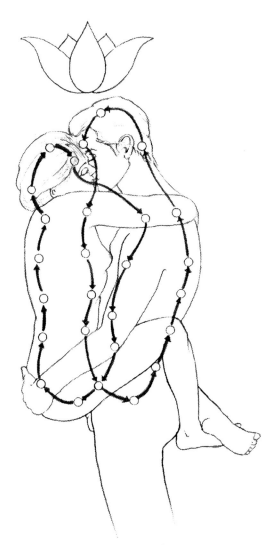

Lovers sharing in-jaculation

Energetic Orgasms

There is a point in your evolutionary development where orgasms move beyond physical, physiological experiences and into the next level–orgasms of your energy systems. Energy-system orgasms still involve the anatomy and all other aspects of physical orgasms, but more is added. Now you can take conscious control of physical stimulation and excitation and channel it throughout your body. Now you can control the sexual energy that ordinarily moves down and out of the body and redirect it inward and upward for rejuvenation and more advanced forms of orgasm.

EXERCISE:

Advanced In-jaculation

Once again, the success of practicing in-jaculation is in proportion to your ability to gain control over your PC muscle and to understand your body's physiology well enough to recognize the signs of an impending orgasm. This foreknowledge gives you the time to shift your orgasm into an in-jaculation before you reach the point of no return. This exercise is applicable for men and women.

1. Sit comfortably with your back straight and your feet flat on the floor.

2. Draw your attention to the ovaries (women) or testicles (men). Then, rub them with your fingertips until they feel like they are becoming warm. Also, mentally assist the rubbing by visualizing the warming of the ovaries and testicles.

3. When you feel a sensation of warmth or tingling in the glands (ovaries or testicles), take a quick inhalation and draw the energy from the glands into the genitals (vagina or penis). Repeat this step several times.

4. Visualize holding the energy in the genitals and gently squeezing the muscles found in that area, while bringing part of your attention back to the glands to gather more energy. Then, on the next inhale, draw another deep breath and bring the energy of the glands into the genitals (as before) but continue drawing it down and around to the tailbone and up to the sacrum (just above the tailbone). Repeat the process of pulling energy from the glands to the tailbone several times before continuing.

5. Begin pumping the sacrum by tightening the Kegel/PC muscle and then relaxing it–but only half way. Tighten again and relax half way again. This contracting of the PC muscle will assist in pumping energy up the spine. Be sure to mentally assist the flow of energy by visualizing its movement.

6. Take long deep breaths as you pump the sacrum and draw the energy from the glands all the way down to the tailbone and up the spine to the base of the neck, where the neck and shoulders join. Repeat this six times.

7. Similar to the last step, take long deep breaths as you pump the sacrum and draw the energy from the glands to the tailbone and up the spine to the base of the skull at the top of the neck. Repeat this six times.

8. Once again, take long deep breaths as you pump the sacrum and draw the energy from the glands down to the tailbone and up the spine to the top of the head. Repeat this six times. After the next repetition, relax and feel the energy, from a single point at the top of the head, spiraling outward to the universe. Open your consciousness to the experience of timelessness. When you feel that the exercise is complete, spiral the energy back into the top of your head on an inhalation.

9. Now, touch your tongue to the top of your mouth, take a deep breath and, as you exhale, visualize and feel the energy at the top of your head slowly pouring downward through the middle of your face, past your throat chakra, and filling your heart center. Repeat this a few times.

10. As energy fills your heart chakra, let your mind fill with thoughts of love and compassion. Then, after a couple of minutes, extend this energy of love to yourself and others in the form of a brief prayer.

11. Finally, take a long deep breath as you pump the sacrum and draw the energy from the ovaries/testicles, down to the tailbone, and then up the spine to the base of the neck, and to the top of the head. As you exhale, allow the energy to flow down the front of your body, past your heart center, and into your navel center (which is located two inches below your navel). Visualize the energy swirling there. Place your hands over this center and gently rub. The energy will be stored here for the body to use as vitality in the future. Repeat this six times.

EXERCISE:

Energy Orgasm

It can take time for some people to experience results in awakening energetic orgasms. Being able to feel an energetic orgasm depends greatly on your ability to sense and visualize energy and your willingness to breathe and moan erotically. Yet, as you learn to delay orgasms and develop proper breathing and energy movement, you are preparing your systems for an enhanced orgasmic experience. You are healing and clearing physical, energetic, and emotional blocks. This healing and clearing of blockages frees up space for a greater quantity and quality of orgasmic energy to move throughout your body.

1. Lie back on a comfortable, but firm, surface and begin taking a few relaxing breaths. Empty your mind.

2. Begin taking in slow, circular breaths; inhaling through your nose and exhaling through your mouth, with no pauses in between breaths.

3. On the inhale, rock your pelvis by arching your lower back. Then, exhale and flatten your lower back. Also, as you exhale, squeeze your PC muscle, thus stimulating the clitoris and G-spot or the penis and prostate, while simultaneously pumping energy upward and throughout your body.

4. Let the breathing and contractions be sensual and erotic. Rub your chest and nipples and make moaning sounds.

5. Imagine that as you are contracting your PC muscle, you are drawing energy into your genitals.

6. Channel this energy upward to each chakra along your spine until you reach the crown center at the top of your head.

7. When the energy reaches your head, imagine a fountain of ecstatic light blasting out into the universe. After a few moments, become aware of all of your chakras radiating and receiving light energy.

8. You may soon feel an energetic orgasm. Relax and let it happen. If you make any attempt to force or control it, you will prevent the experience from occurring.

CHAPTER 5

Your Emotions

The Effects of Your First Sexual Experiences

The emotional effects of our earliest sexual experiences are so powerful that they permanently impact our future sexual choices. In many respects, our earliest sexual experiences remain with us for the rest of our lives. For some, the first sexual experience was loving, romantic, and/or educational. For others, the encounter was vastly different. Whether positive or negative, these early events experienced as children, teenagers, or adults determine what our relationships will become. They affect our ability to choose healthy, responsible partners. Nevertheless, whatever unhealthy patterns may have driven us in the past, sexual healing is possible and will assist in the breaking of these patterns that "the experts" predict will remain with us permanently.

Most people acquire sexual inhibitions at some point in their lives. A few of these are conscious, but many are not. Most inhibitions arise from religious conditioning, parental attitudes or traumatic experiences.

Everyone would benefit from taking time to do a self-inventory, especially in relation to the life-long effects of their sexual experiences. The effects of such experiences are usually underestimated, but it's clear to most counselors and practitioners of sacred sexuality that these events have profound effects on their clients (and their lives)–from the depths of their psyches to the cells of their bodies.

Responsibility and Boundaries

Emotions are an important bridge between the physical and spiritual worlds, as well as between physical and soul-level (total-being) orgasms. The unresolved issues within your emotional being need not be healed and perfect, but they certainly must be in the process of *heal-ing*. If left unchecked, your unhealed emotional wounds will act as a barrier to *safety*. Without a feeling of safety, you cannot *trust* totally. Without trust, you cannot experience sacred sexuality and the total-being orgasms that are an integral part of any sacred sexual experience.

If you desire the most amazing sexual experience possible, you need to accept responsibility for creating a safe and tangible connection with God, yourself, and others. You also need to be responsible for doing personal healing work because this work will enable you to create healthier boundaries in your life and with your lovers.

The concept of setting boundaries has often been misrepresented to mean learning how to say "no!" Yet, this is not the case. **Having clear boundaries means that you are in touch enough with the healthy, loving part of yourself to know what does and doesn't work for your higher good and to choose accordingly.** To establish clear boundaries successfully and consistently requires a sense of self-love and self-worth.

As you develop a clearer sense of responsibility and boundaries, you will increase your ability to create relationships wherein you feel enough trust and comfort to openly communicate and heal all that would otherwise keep you from experiencing a life of passion and bliss.

Dealing with Inhibitions

Some people have very serious, justifiable reasons for their sexual inhibitions. Nevertheless, repression of their sexuality is not their natural state of being, nor is it meant to be permanent. With enough courage, anyone and everyone can heal. Healing sexual inhibitions requires pushing through personal issues in this area. For instance, some people are inhibited about the use of sexual terminology. Yet how is it possible for people to be truly comfortable with sexual activity if they aren't even comfortable with the terms describing those activities? For example, **did you know that the original purpose (and meaning) for the word "FUCK" derived from a legal mandate that allowed a person to <u>F</u>ornicate <u>U</u>nder the <u>C</u>onsent of the <u>K</u>ing?** It's true! Most of the terminology surrounding sex has a meaningful history. But these meanings were forgotten, and people (who were probably sexually inhibited) began to assign "naughty," negative connotations to these words.

Most of our inhibitions and belief systems (especially those unconsciously chosen) come from our parents, friends, culture, religion, and past experiences. They rarely arise from conscious, clear decisions in the present moment, but instead arise from old, learned patterns. This fact applies to both men and women. Men, for example, are brought up to view almost everything associated with girls as negative. If a boy is perceived as weak, his peers tauntingly call him a *"girl."* Since emotions are archetypically feminine, if a male detaches from his femininity, he also cuts off from feeling. **Symbolically, men cut off from their hearts and emotions by wearing ties around their necks and detach from their bodies by wearing belts around their waists.**

The deepest layer of emotional issues or inhibitions has to do with core feelings and beliefs. Most core issues develop during the first few years of life and unconsciously influence our sense of identity. Patterns associated with core issues and unconscious belief systems usually make our decisions *for* us. Of course, this conditioning can change if we do a self-inventory and begin a healing process. We are then free to adopt our own opinions–those based on current feelings and inspirations. This freedom gradually results in our letting go and allowing our "true self" to come to life and playfully express the feelings of our hearts.

Remember, the experience of sacred sexuality requires the ability to relax and let go–to free our minds of extraneous thoughts and our bodies of inhibition and tension. It also requires releasing any sensual sounds evoked during arousal and expressing them without inhibitions.

Healing Sexual Trauma

What is sexual trauma? How do you know if the term applies to you? For people who have been raped or molested, the answers to these questions are usually obvious. However, **sexual trauma can also include being shamed, having abortions, repressing guilt about past sexual behavior, and**

feeling conflict over religious, social or family beliefs or ethics. Basically, any experience that lacks love's presence is traumatic to the heart and soul and therefore affects your life and body.

Traumas or inhibitions can block the neurotransmitters from the genitals to the brain—even to the point, for example, where a woman can physically experience vaginal contractions that simulate an orgasm, *but* her brain receives no signals of pleasure.

In such instances, sexual healing techniques can effect a reprogramming of some of these blocked channels. Once new levels of love and trust are imprinted, the woman's yoni can respond with deeper levels of release and orgasm. When healing takes place, the woman's pleasure-signals can move unimpeded to her brain, enabling her to orgasm more easily.

Additionally, trauma and inhibitions can show up as a loss of sensation in the yoni (for a woman) or some forms of erectile dysfunction (for a man). Successful healing can be assisted, in some cases, by massaging the wounded (numb or painful) region with a slow, light, healing touch, while the recipient breathes as deeply and calmly as possible and remains present.

When your partner is sexually wounded and you are encouraging healing, you are, in effect, asking her (or him) to surrender to a level of trust and freedom that might be new to her. For this reason, it is imperative to gain your partner's trust. **You can earn trust by demonstrating that your partner's well-being, and not just the activity of sex, is your primary goal.** You can also gain trust by being in tune with your partner—body and soul.

Sexual Disorders

Sexual dysfunction usually surfaces in one of a few specific forms that differ from a man to a woman. For a male, sexual dysfunction can manifest as impotence or premature ejaculation. For a female, it usually manifests as the inability to orgasm.

Sexual trauma results in feelings and memories becoming trapped in the body and causing sexual dysfunction. These traumas also often result in some form of sexual "acting out." Unfortunately, this reaction to inner wounds can manifest in the polarity of either sexual starvation *or* sexual overindulgence. Each extreme has its own set of symptoms. The topics of sexual trauma and sexual dysfunction are covered more extensively in previous and subsequent sections of this book.

STARVATION:

- ❏ I avoid being sexually attractive.
- ❏ I assume that partners only want me for sex.
- ❏ I resist sexual contact ranging from kissing to intercourse.
- ❏ I experience shame about my body and/or past experiences.
- ❏ I continue the above patterns even if my life suffers.

OVERINDULGENCE:

- ❏ I pursue high-risk sex.
- ❏ I have sex with people even when I am not attracted to them.
- ❏ I obsess about sex and think about getting people into bed.
- ❏ I use sex to manage my physical and/or emotional health.
- ❏ I continue the above patterns even if my life suffers.

Emotional Orgasms

As we heal from sexual traumas and inhibitions, our bodies and souls begin to feel liberated and therefore exhibit signs of letting go. This releasing can manifest in various types of orgasms–including emotional orgasms.

The best way to define emotional orgasms is to start by dividing them into two types. First, there can be moments of spontaneous emotional release expressed as panic or tears during the lovemaking experience. This type of emotional orgasm can also result in laughter, which is another way to release physical, energetic, and emotional tensions. Such symptoms indicate the surfacing of old, buried emotional traumas–even without conscious visions or memories. The releasing of these intense emotions is a form of orgasm.

Despite their unpredictable onset and awkward timing (as well as any helplessness felt by either partner), these releases are very healing. After every emotional release, time should be taken for deep, calming breaths, while the person releasing focuses on, or connects with, the Spiritual Presence of Divine Love and safety.

The second type of emotional orgasm can be triggered by the relief and gratitude partners feel when realizing on some level that they are safe and healing. **This type of emotional orgasm can also be triggered solely by the deep, romantic connection felt by the partners who are sharing the**

experience of lovemaking. These are tears of joy that result from the realization of the depths of love the partners feel for each other.

One way for lovers to experience an emotional orgasm is to create a deep level of connection through slow body movements and deep eye contact. When making love, gaze into each other's eyes as much as possible. If there is truly a loving intent between lovers, the two of them will notice a deepening of vulnerability and love. Eye-to-eye contact will dissolve the false masks that prevent true intimacy. So, lock eyes, kiss often, and verbally communicate by sharing your deepest feelings. There is a possibility that connecting this deeply with your current partner may feel uncomfortable. So don't force it! If you give it a try, you might discover that it proves healing to you both. But if you cannot do this exercise, you might need to consider why you are making love to someone with whom you cannot even make eye contact.

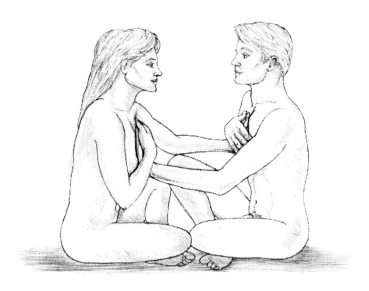

Connecting eye to eye with your partner

TECHNIQUE:

Connecting Eye to Eye

The following is a common Sufi exercise used for creating a connection between two or more people. This exercise, which is especially good for creating a connection between lovers, can be done clothed or naked.

STEP 1: Sit cross-legged facing your partner with knees touching.

STEP 2: Each of you place your right palm on your partner's heart chakra and your left hand over his or her right hand on your own chest.

STEP 3: Gaze with love and compassion into each other's eyes and synchronize your breathing.

STEP 4: Feel the loving connection between you. Send loving energy from your heart, through your right hand, and into your partner's heart.

STEP 5: Draw the loving, heart energy of your partner into your left hand and to your heart, completing a full cycle from heart to heart. Then continue this loving cycle back and forth several times, absorbing the feeling of connectedness.

STEP 6: As you feel a deepening sense of connection, begin imagining that you are seeing beyond the human body of your partner and envisioning his or her divine, god and goddess self.

STEP 7: Finally, when you both feel a sense of completion, give thanks to each other.

CHAPTER 6

Your Mind

How It All Began

As previously mentioned, it's easy (and all too convenient) to underestimate the effect your early life has had on who you are today. This inclination holds true especially for sexual influences–particularly, a person's *first* sexual experience. Take a moment to review the following questions and freely journal whatever answers come up.

Once you complete these checklists, take time to journal and do a self-inventory to discover what kinds of emotions have been evoked.

❏ How did you first learn about sex?

❏ Did you play sexual games as a child? What were they like and how did you feel?

❏ When did you first learn to masturbate? What was it like and how did you feel?

❏ As an adolescent, what was your general attitude or feeling about sex?

❏ What were your parent's views on sex?

My Attitudes About Sex

Sometimes it's hard to separate concepts of healthy, from unhealthy, sex. This lack of clarity can result from confusion concerning your known or unknown attitudes about sex. Take another moment to review these questions to see where you stand in your attitudes about sex. Check the boxes that feel like an accurate description of *your* experiences or viewpoints. Then write down your thoughts and feelings about each topic as they arise.

- ☐ Sex feels like an obligation or duty.
- ☐ Sex is something I do to get something else.
- ☐ It's okay for only one partner to enjoy sex.
- ☐ My parents demonstrated healthy intimacy and affection with each other.
- ☐ Sex feels dirty to me.
- ☐ I am comfortable using basic sex toys (such as vibrators and dildos).
- ☐ I am uncomfortable using basic sex toys (such as vibrators and dildos).
- ☐ I sometimes leave my body during sex.
- ☐ Sex feels scary to me.
- ☐ Sex feels secretive to me.
- ☐ I feel satisfied with the experience when I have sex.
- ☐ I feel unsatisfied with the experience when I have sex.
- ☐ I equate sex with sexual abuse.
- ☐ Sex is an escape.
- ☐ Sex is humiliating to me or others.
- ☐ I feel addicted to sex.
- ☐ I sometimes have dark thoughts, fantasies or embarrassing sexual fetishes.
- ☐ Sex can be used to get love or to feel loved.
- ☐ Sex makes me feel like I'm losing control.
- ☐ I have noticed an attraction for the same gender.
- ☐ Sex is hurtful or painful.
- ☐ I use sex for power and control.
- ☐ Sex benefits men more than women.
- ☐ Sex is a lower, base expression.
- ☐ Males have a right to demand sex from their partners.
- ☐ Sex is used for expressing dark fantasies.
- ☐ Sex is uncomfortable for me.
- ☐ When having sex, I only get turned on if I fantasize about something else.

My Self Image

Sexual confusion can influence how you feel about yourself and your sexuality. Take a moment to review these questions to see where you are in your attitudes about your sexual self. Then write whatever comes up concerning these topics.

- ❏ I don't like my body.
- ❏ I feel as though there is something wrong with me sexually.
- ❏ I am confused about my sexual orientation.
- ❏ I'm afraid of what emotions will arise if I let myself go–sexually.
- ❏ I give in too quickly or easily to sex.
- ❏ I feel like a victim in sex.
- ❏ I feel sexually inadequate.
- ❏ I don't like parts of my sexual anatomy.
- ❏ I would like to improve myself as a sexual person.
- ❏ I would like to improve upon my reactions to touch and sex.
- ❏ I have made unhealthy (or high risk) choices with my sexual practices.

Indulging Your Fantasies

Basically, there are two types of sexual fantasizing. The first involves mental imagery, and the second includes role-play. Both of them rely heavily on imagination. One of the benefits of utilizing either form of fantasy is that it can evoke orgasms via mental stimulation. Fantasies can also create a more adventurous lovemaking experience.

As already mentioned, the latter form of fantasy involves acting out through role-play. This fantasy can include anything from dressing up in costumes to various forms of bondage. Some couples like to play such role-games as having the male pretend to be a stranger, sweep the woman off her feet, and then make passionate love to her. Other partners become aroused by going to bars or restaurants and pretending to be strangers, so they can flirt with others. Then they finally "make a move" for each other.

Fantasizing is not illicit behavior. Its unfortunate negative reputation

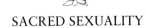

comes from its being such a secret part of our world. When we have to hide our sexuality, it becomes a "skeleton in the closet" and takes on a cloud of shame. **The same gift of fantasizing can be used by a sexually healthy person to increase arousal, or it can drag a sex addict into uncontrollable behaviors.** The former is natural, but the latter is often the result of sexual repression and/or trauma.

Some individuals find themselves fantasizing about other lovers while having sex with a current partner. Although this need not be seen as "wrong," it certainly inhibits being fully present. So, one of the best solutions is to share your fantasies with your partner (unless of course it is not appropriate, as when you are fantasizing about someone else). Your partner can learn to use your fantasies to increase your arousal during lovemaking, allowing you to integrate your mind with your body and soul.

Some women who have been raped find that in order to get turned on or have an orgasm, they have to fantasize (mentally or through acting out) the intensity of the rape. Once again, this fantasy or acting out is not "bad." It's simply one way of trying to recreate the event in an attempt to come to terms with it. Of course these women will not succeed in healing through repetitively acting out. They need to mend their wounds through therapy and sexual healing.

Mental Orgasms

Mental orgasms can best be defined as orgasms that are reached either exclusively with images held in the mind *or* with the assistance of concentrated visualization. In the first example, the mind enhances physical stimulation, even to the point of an orgasmic release. In fact, many of the arts of sacred sexuality promote the use of the mind to evoke as much excitation as possible. Partners can increase each other's arousal through imagination by the use of erotically stimulating thoughts and words prior to, or instead of, actions.

The second possibility uses concentration and the skill of *projecting* your thoughts to another person for the purpose of sexual arousal. You do not have to be in physical contact with this person to succeed. The person you are thinking about can be on the other side of the room or the other side of the planet, for that matter. Distance is no obstacle! First, your mind can, and must, eliminate any thought or belief that distance is a barrier to oneness. Then, with enough focus, one lover can mentally arouse another—even to the point of orgasm. It helps for your partner to be tuned in to receiving at the same time.

EXERCISE:

Mind Pleasuring

The mind is one of the most powerful tools in lovemaking and sacred sexuality. It's the disciplined mind that enables you to remain centered and focused. It's also the mind that enables you to concentrate enough to connect with your imagination, which is necessary for visualizing the anatomy of your lover. The following exercise is to enhance your ability to mentally connect with your partner.

1. With, or without, your partner being in the same room (but always with his or her consent), practice visualizing your partner sitting in front of you. Say a short prayer asking for Divine Love to guide this exercise.

2. Allow the two separate images of you and your partner to remain distinct, but visualize an etheric energy joining the two of you, as if your auras are merging, but not your bodies. Maintain this image as clearly as possible.

3. Visualize your partner reaching out and touching your heart and sharing a loving comment with you. Follow this by seeing yourself doing the same thing for him or her.

4. Visualize your partner reaching out and touching your genitals with sensual strokes, as the two of you moan in response to the arousal.

5. Now visualize reaching for your partner's genitals and stroking them with the same love you have shared in previous moments of lovemaking. It's essential that you take your time and imagine every detail possible. If you imagine running your fingers across his or her pubic hair, for example, see and feel the hair beneath your fingers, caressing your skin. If you imagine touching your partner's clitoris or penis, visualize running your fingertips across her clitoral head or the ridge around the head of his penis.

6. Raise your partner to a point of orgasm a few times, backing off before he or she cums. Be sure to hear the moans of ecstasy calling for more.

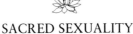

7. Finally, imagine feeling your partner's body arch off the ground as he or she prepares for orgasm. Continue the visualized stimulation seeing your partner explode in pleasure. Hear the deep moans. You might even see your partner having several releases.

8. Now imagine your partner falling into a deep restfulness with energy gently flowing through his or her body from head to toe. Then allow the image to fade as you give thanks for the sharing.

CHAPTER 7

Your Soul

Being Present

Being fully aware of the present moment is one of the most effective ways to access the soul. When experiencing sacred sexuality, you can increase desire and pleasure by anticipating each stroke from your lover. It is important to appreciate and respond to any degree of sensation, no matter how slight. Be conscious of each stroke, movement, sound or fragrance–every sensation of the moment–to access your soul and that of your lover.

When making love, you might be thinking about something else–sexual agendas or something totally unrelated to the present experience. To avoid such distractions, remain focused and feel each sensation, as well as the pleasure you are giving and receiving. If, while making love, you start thinking about performance and its result (rather than being in the present moment), focus on one of the techniques for enhancing the sexual experience to help you return to the present. Once refocused in the moment, forget the techniques. Relax, breathe slowly and gently; go with the natural flow of energy as it unfolds. **You need not force anything. Don't be goal-oriented! Be in the here and now, and feel every sensation, touch, and subtle movement.**

Again, you can intensify pleasure by remaining focused on the present moment and avoid being goal-oriented. Furthermore, the receiving partner should surrender body and soul and remain focused on all orgasmic sensations commencing with (or even before) the first stroke. In other words, the receiving partner should totally yield to his or her partner and surrender to the pleasure being given.

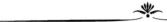

My true self is blossoming. Not by direction or force, just by surrender. And now my sexuality and heart are becoming so merged that I can hardly put my attention on one without exciting the other.

–Valerie Brooks *(Tantric Awakening)*

To know what your partner is feeling, check-in and see how *you* feel. It's uncanny how we mirror each other, and the sexual arena is no exception. Often, when *you* lose concentration, your partner will start to drift away as well. For this reason, be aware of your own feelings and experiences. In fact, if you catch yourself slipping out of the moment, come back before your partner reacts to your lack of presence. Observing your own feelings will also help you to stay present.

Developing Intuitive Skills

Intuition is an attribute of the heart and soul. **As you develop a greater presence of love within your heart and soul, so too will the level of your intuition increase.** Since intuitive awareness is also magnified by the ability to feel oneness with others, healthy relationships offer the perfect environment to develop intuition. This fact can be witnessed in the intuitive connection between a mother and child or between a couple who have been together long enough to nurture this quality.

Intuition is an ideal tool to deepen the sacredness of any sexual experience. You need only be still, hold love as a priority, and sensitively listen to the needs of all involved. For some partners, intuitive sensitivity seems natural, almost second nature. For others, it develops over time. Whichever the case, it's worthwhile to practice exercises that enhance intuitive connectedness.

Accessing the Soul Through the Heart

It is often said that the eyes are the windows to the soul. This saying becomes vividly true when you are sitting in the sacred presence of a partner, gazing into his or her eyes, breathing together, toning or praying, and sharing secrets from the heart and soul. It is also powerful to gaze into your own eyes while looking in a mirror.

EXERCISE:

Gazing Into Your Soul

The idea of gazing into your own eyes in a mirror may at first sound absurd. But before you scoff at the idea, take a moment to try it. If you practice this exercise with even the slightest sincerity, you may discover, to your surprise, that there are unhealed feelings just below the surface.

1. Find a private room with a large, clean mirror (preferably large enough to see your whole body). Light several candles.
2. Gaze at yourself in the mirror and carefully observe what you see.
3. When finished observing your face and body, look into your eyes and speak to your soul. Tell your soul you are sorry for any ways you have abused or neglected it. Then tell your soul how much you love it and what you will do to nurture it to full maturity.
4. Next, close your eyes and pray to be given the spiritual vision of unconditional love. Then open your eyes and again look carefully at yourself. You might notice different things than you had before, or perhaps you'll see the same things but feel differently about them. Some individuals find that using the prayed-for vision of the soul (spiritual vision) gives them the ability to see auras–including their own in the mirror.
5. After you complete the dialog with your soul, give thanks to it for its beauty. Then give thanks to God for blessing you with rebirth.

Soul-Level (Total-Being) Orgasms

Physiologically speaking, an orgasm is a build-up of sexual *fluids* waiting to be released upon climax. A soul-level orgasm, on the other hand, is a

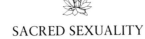

build-up of *energy* waiting to be released at the moment of surrendering to love's presence.

A soul-level orgasm occurs in one of two ways. The first way involves the building up of a physical, energetic, emotional, and spiritual connection until all sensation of the body disappears and the soul rises to the foreground. The second way to experience a soul-level orgasm is through the build up of spiritual, energetic ecstasy to the extent that physical touch becomes unnecessary to achieve the orgasm. The latter way includes spiritual ecstatic experiences where a person rides waves of ecstasy that can take him or her into dimensions of the soul.

Energetic ecstasy and soul-level orgasms occur when a spiritual frequency or vibration reaches down and stimulates, or caresses, a person's body (nervous system) and soul (heart-center), resulting in an ecstatic experience within the body. Although the body *can* be manually stimulated (without spiritual integrity or intent) to the point of creating an energetic (and *seemingly* ecstatic) response, this purely physiological experience cannot duplicate the feeling of complete oneness resulting from a soul-level orgasm.

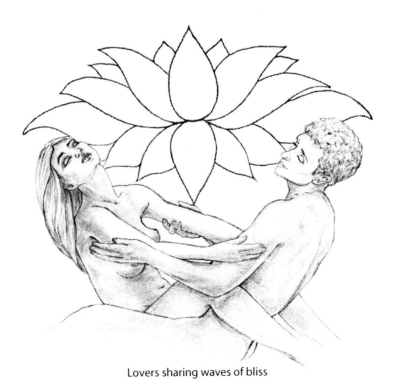

Lovers sharing waves of bliss

142

TECHNIQUE:
Soul-Level (Total-Being) Orgasms

Although some people are fortunate enough to experience a soul-level orgasm with relative ease, such is not the case for most. Instead, most individuals must first acquire the essential ingredients that include feelings of love and trust and the ability to relax totally. Other necessary ingredients are long-term pleasuring and stimulation, plus the time it takes to progress through some of the other, lower levels of orgasm. Provided they are given enough time and pleasuring, a soul-level orgasm is more common for women than men. Their bodies are already tuned-in to the nature of deeper experiences.

Some learned men...say that women...should not study the Kama Sutra. But...this objection does not hold, for women already know the principles of Kama Sutra.

–Kama Sutra

The surest way to create a soul-level orgasm is to be pleasured at length and brought to the point of orgasm at least five to ten times without ejaculation or climaxing. Instead of an ejaculation, practice in-jaculation (channeling the energy upward through the body) and detumescing (calming or stabilizing) the ecstatic energy. Also, combine breath-work, visualization, touch, and soul-to-soul connection to evoke a sensual, energetic response. Then, spread this energy throughout the body as if it were a fuel awaiting the proper moment to be ignited. Once ignited (through proper stimulation), the orgasm, which usually originates in the genitals, will spread like a wildfire throughout the body and build into a full-body, total-being orgasm.

This level of orgasm builds until the whole body starts to vibrate, hence the name "total-being orgasm." At other times, the order of sensations is reversed; the body vibrates first and then calms into deep, orgasmic waves. When a soul-level orgasm builds up enough energy, it blasts through all the chakras and energy systems, producing an even more dramatic, ecstatic experience.

This buildup of energy can be accomplished while being manually or orally pleasured *or* during intercourse. Doing so while having intercourse can prove more difficult from the potentially distracting body positioning and mutual stimulation. On the other hand, building up energy while being pleasured simply involves receiving and surrendering. This lack of effort frees the body to experience greater releases.

For a man to experience a total-being orgasm, he must learn to override, or control, all automatic ejaculatory reactions, such as body tensing. Ejaculation must become a conscious choice. Achieving this goal initially involves completely giving in to all sensations of pleasure and stimulation, while relaxing the PC muscle, the anal sphincter, and the "smooth muscles" around the urethra.

To further develop ejaculatory control, the male's partner can stimulate his penis, while paying close attention to his inner and outer reactions. She can seduce, tease, and entice him–again and again. Thus, she can excite him, build his energy, pause prior to orgasm, and then continue to increase his level of arousal. Finally, before an orgasmic release, both parties can relax momentarily. She can lighten her touch while they both mentally disperse the energy throughout his body.

Since there is no one, single way to achieve the experience of soul-level, total-being orgasms, the following are suggested steps to assist you. You may find a favorite solo exercise does the trick for you. Partners are encouraged to use any of the manual and/or oral pleasuring and lovemaking techniques. Any of these may be the right one for you and your partner. Whatever techniques you use should be incorporated into the following additional steps.

STEP 1: Practice living a healthier life. Take the proper nutrients and supplements, and practice exercises to open any blocks in the muscles and energy systems.

STEP 2: Take a personal inventory focused on your past sexual issues and experiences. Consult a counselor or sex therapist if needed.

STEP 3: Create a loving and safe environment for self-pleasuring, pleasuring from your partner or for lovemaking. Being in the presence of love makes the difference between having an orgasm that is merely energetic and one that reaches the soul level.

STEP 4: Use as many pillows as is necessary to create a feeling of floating, allowing all the muscles to relax completely.

STEP 5: Take time for prayer and for connecting with your partner, if one is present.

STEP 6: Choose a form of stimulation that works best for you, and plan on receiving for at least half an hour to one hour. Rid your mind of any thoughts of rushing or concerns that you are failing because it isn't happening in the timeframe you'd prefer. The process must be given plenty of time. It may even take days of practicing.

STEP 7: When you feel arousal, it's important to let the feeling expand throughout your body by not tensing and by releasing deep moans.

STEP 8: Imagine that you are floating and that the pleasure you are receiving is not just in your genitals, but includes your entire body. The more you see and feel your body as one whole unit, the greater the likelihood it will respond as such.

STEP 9: Do not reach for an orgasm or ejaculation. Instead, let each sensation be a total body experience. Eventually, you will discover that even the slightest pleasure becomes a joy-filled dance with the universe.

CHAPTER 8

Your Spirit

Entering the Holy of Holies

Once upon a time, we experienced the Garden of Eden. When we lost site of living in bliss (and departed from paradise), we were told that an angel, with a "sword of light," would guard the gates of the Garden. Ancient mystery schools teach that as we re-approach the threshold of the proverbial paradise, we will be met with a vision of this same light. The quest to return to the Garden of Eden is ages old. To return to Eden is to discover the Holy Grail or the Ark of the Covenant. Yet we have found that Eden, like Heaven, is not a place but a "state of mind."

Once our consciousness is re-attuned to this blissful level of being, an orgasm within the upper chakras and the brain takes place, referred to as a "spiritual orgasm." It is described in detail in the tantric teachings of Buddha. The techniques and their effects for experiencing physical and energetic orgasms (previously discussed in this material) are merely preparations for attaining the supreme experienc of spiritual orgasms. Ultimately, the practice and process of attaining spiritual orgasms are not dependent upon actual sexual contact. The primary purpose of practicing sacred sexuality has always been to achieve union, or a blissful dance with the Divine. Having now attained such union through spiritual orgasms, our consciousness is swept away into a sea of bliss unlike any that accompanies sexual orgasms. This bliss doesn't pass away with time but remains permanently encoded in our hearts and souls.

Most of the exercises related to spiritual orgasms are done in the mind and *not* with the body. Nonetheless, the effects are felt, seen, and heard in body, mind, and soul.

Revelation...reflects the original form of communication between God and His creation, involving the extremely personal sense of creation sometimes saught in physical relationships. Physical closeness cannot achieve it.

—A Course in Miracles

Spiritual Orgasms

Of the few primary practices that lead to the experiencing of a spiritual orgasm, none can replace the daily practice and application of communing with God and living a life of loving service. A spiritual orgasm is a spiritual and physiological process that first takes place within the skull of your head and then fills your body. Practicing advanced forms of meditation, breath-work, and in-jaculations are all valid ways to *assist* the process of a spiritual orgasm. Such exercises include the cobra breath (learned in Kriya or Tantric yoga), a technique never written down but only passed down through initiations between teacher and student. The cobra breath clears the etheric pathways within the *sushumna* (spinal) meridian. The vacuum created by this cleansing clears the way for energy and spinal fluid to rise from the sacrum and to the brain. The profound effects of true communion with God are not unknown to highly evolved mystics, Tibetan Buddhists, and advanced practitioners of meditation.

By regularly communing with God through meditation, you activate a tone, or vibrational frequency, at the center of your head. This (often imperceptible) tone awakens the kundalini energy (or *sushumna*) *and* cerebral spinal fluid at the base of the spine, beckoning it upward along the spine and then to the brain. At this point, cerebral spinal fluid fills the inside of the skull (cranium), creating an energy-grid between the two hemispheres of the brain. This total-brain awakening also activates the sphenoid bone of the cranium, which, in turn, stimulates the hypothalamus and the pineal and pituitary glands. Then these glands send messages of love and healing, as well as orgasmic-light sensations, to other major glands and throughout your body.

Stimulation of the pituitary and pineal glands also creates an arc of light that illuminates your entire brain and skull (a part of the body that Taoists refer to as the "Original Cavity" or "Ancestral Hall"). This light-activation, results in the awakening of your mind's eye and your crown chakra, blasting energy up into the heavens. This liquid-light then pours over your forehead and down the front of your body, a process well described in the 23rd Psalm of the Bible which reads, "Thou hast anointed my head with oil; my cup runneth over...I will dwell in the house of the Lord forever."

EXERCISE:
Ecstatic Meditation

Although it is almost impossible to describe the experience or effects of a spiritual orgasm, the most common examples of this level of orgasm are either the ecstatic trance-like state of a spiritual visionary or the deep levels of meditation attained by living masters. The effects of spiritual ecstasy are so profound that many masters who experience this level of consciousness no longer use the body as a tool for energy enhancement–Spirit, in itself, becomes sufficient. Consequently, once this level of consciousness is attained, there is a temptation to ignore and neglect the body and one's material, personal life. This highly evolved path is appropriate only for a few select individuals whose constant spiritual focus is directed exclusively toward maintaining harmony on the planet. For most people, however, there needs to be a balance between the attainment of spiritual mastery and the honoring of one's humanness. Living this balance between the human and the divine is the most challenging of all lessons or initiations.

STEP 1: Sit comfortably and draw in slow, deep breaths. As you breathe deeply, expand your entire torso. With the first two or three inhalations, let your torso expand *forward*. With the next inhalations, see and feel your upper and lower back expanding *backward*. Then, with the next couple of inhalations, let your sides expand *outward*. Finally, with the next inhalations, let your diaphragm and solar plexus push *downward* towards your tailbone. Relax all your limbs, as well as your torso, and feel your entire body breathing in harmony.

STEP 2: Acknowledge your desire to surrender all aspects of your life and being to God. Also surrender all control of your body.

STEP 3: Turn your eyes upwards, toward your forehead, and imagine a

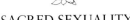

point of light in the center of your head directly behind your third eye.

STEP 4: Concentrate on a mantra, such as "universal love " or "Divine Presence."

STEP 5: Remain focused on your mantra. If other thoughts or feelings arise, allow them to pass as you inhale deeply. Simultaneously repeat your mantra, quietly to yourself. On your exhalation, mentally repeat the words, "And so it is." Use this re-focusing discipline as needed.

STEP 6: After maintaining a focus on your mantra for several minutes, consciously surrender to the meaning of the mantra. Ask God what it's like to *feel* universal love or to be *filled* with Divine Presence. Then surrender to the answer.

STEP 7: With consistent practice, you will pass through several stages of spiritual orgasm. The first stage evokes a feeling of calmness and centeredness. The second stage begins the "light-show," where you may see a brilliant white light (or perhaps sparkles) filling your head. This light and its accompanying feeling will inevitably expand to fill your body. The third stage of spiritual orgasm takes you to (and beyond) the light that draws you to the gates of Eden. Now you *enter* the Garden and begin feeling, experiencing, and integrating all that the Garden represents. At this stage, you become a "light unto the world."

STEP 8: The final stage of spiritual orgasm is not "final" at all, but a constant cycle of integration and application. Apply what you gain, and more will be given.

"In Sutra alone (the fundamental teachings of Buddha) there is no liberation. The Highest Yoga Tantra teachings are Buddha's ultimate intention."

–*Mahamudra Tantra*
(Geshe Kelsang Gyatso)

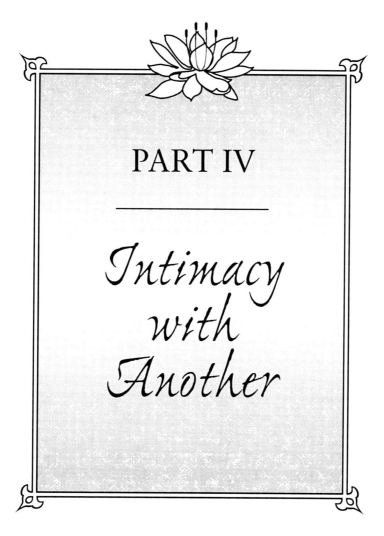

PART IV

Intimacy with Another

Foreplay

Foreplay is, as the word implies, play-fullness before intercourse. Therefore, it should be experienced as such–fun and spontaneous, yet enhanced by tools and techniques to stimulate arousal. Remember, though, that the deep *connection* between partners, moreso than technique, is the greatest aphrodisiac. So maintain a connection to your own heart and soul with the intent of remaining connected to your partner's heart and soul as well. Be sure to draw from imagination and spontaneity as the foundation for your tools of foreplay. But, most important, take your time.

It's been said that women fake orgasms because men fake foreplay. Arousing a woman is different from arousing a man. A woman needs time. Foreplay in general, should be slow and lighthearted, rather than rushed or excessively stimulating. If you rush and overstimulate a man, he can suffer premature ejaculation. Overstimulating a woman can result in excessive excitation in her clitoris or G-spot, thus preventing the relaxation necessary for the deepest levels of orgasm.

The word foreplay has erroneously taken on the negative connotation of sexually stimulating acts for the sole purpose of achieving intercourse. In truth, foreplay can be a sensual, sexual experience in and of itself–without necessarily progressing to intercourse. Yet, foreplay can certainly be followed by intercourse. In fact, foreplay is so important that it should nearly always be a part of intercourse. Still, foreplay is not dependent upon intercourse.

Playful teasing is an invaluable part of foreplay. Teasing involves enticing your partner onward, offering suggestions of promised delights that draw him or her closer, and then easing off slightly. Effective teasing requires an awareness of the energy level between you and your partner, noticing when the optimum sensations have been reached and then knowing when it is time to back off. Teasing is not a means of controlling your partner, nor is it meant to deny your partner pleasure. Instead, teasing is a means of heightening your partner's arousal and intensifying his or her sensual enjoyment.

Traditionally, the Tantric ritual for lovers begins with the partners symbolically purifying their bodies by washing or bathing each other. Next, lovers connect heart-to-heart by breathing together and exchanging kind words. Then, they connect soul-to-soul by praying together.

In addition to the rituals of cleansing and connecting, lovers have many other activities to choose from during their initial stages of lovemaking. The repertoire of foreplay is far greater than genital stimulation in preparation for intercourse. The choices can include any combination of the list below.

1. Creating Environment (Chapter 9)
2. Cleansing (Chapter 10)
3. Communicating and Connecting (Chapter 11)
4. Kissing and Mouth-play (Chapter 12)
5. Massaging and Caressing (Chapter 13)
6. Oral Sex (Chapter 14)

Initial Contact

The *Kama Sutra* is specific about the art of embracing or making physical contact. It begins by dividing initial physical contact into two groups, each with four types of contact, for a total of eight. The first four types of embrace are for the purpose of initial contact. These are as follows:

1. *The Touching Embraces*–a purposeful, gentle groping, goosing or stroking that says, "I want you."
2. *The Piercing Embrace*–a woman brushes her breasts against a man, and he responds by grabbing the breasts with conviction.
3. *The Rubbing Embrace*–a couple rubs against each other while they stand or walk together.
4. *The Pressing Embrace*–one partner pins the other against a wall with his (or her) body.

Any one, or more, of the above-mentioned embraces could progress into the second set of four, which include the following:

1. *The Embrace of The Twining of a Vine*–the woman takes one of the first four types of embrace to the next level by initiating a more committed form of contact. She stands facing her mate with one leg wrapped around him, while placing one hand behind his head or neck to keep his gaze on her.
2. *The Embrace of Climbing A Tree*–the women stands close to her

partner, places her hands on his shoulders, and raises one leg upon his hip as if she intends to climb on him.

3. *The Embrace or Mixing of Milk and Water*–the woman sits on her partner's lap, while they breathe together and gently embrace with their entire bodies.

4. *The Embrace of Mixing Sesame Seed and Rice*–two lovers lie together and embrace so firmly that all their arms and legs are entwined, maximizing skin-to-skin contact.

CHAPTER 9

The Environment and Setting The Mood

Getting Things Ready

Before a sacred sexual encounter, prepare the room that will become your love chamber. Place any necessary supplies close-by *before* you get started, so there will be fewer distractions and less effort for you and your lover, allowing a fuller surrender to the sensations of the moment. Advanced preparation also includes having an empty stomach, colon, and bladder.

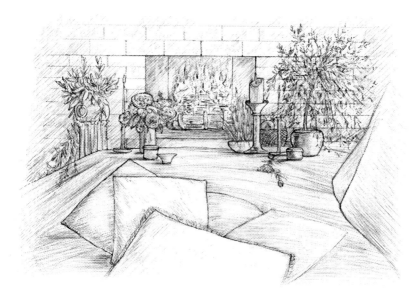

Preparing the environment for love-making

This sacred space we create enhances the mood. It heats up my body, and I feel like I am in a trance. I can close my eyes and a blissful, dreamlike state washes over me–not sleeping, not awake I forget all my problems and flaws and dive into this idyllic dream of sweat and wetness that is too good to believe.

–Valerie Brooks *(Tantric Awakening)*

The undressing of yourself, or each other, can be done at any time during the initial stages of foreplay. Undressing might be included in the early stage of "creating the environment" or during a later part of foreplay, such as "massaging and connecting." **Whenever you choose to unbutton your partner's shirt or blouse or remove his or her pants, remember that you are symbolically disrobing your partner's defenses and exposing the soul.**

Prayer and Meditation

There is no better way to set the desired tone for an intimate encounter than to clearly communicate your intentions and to use some form of spiritual connecting. This communing and connecting might include praying and/or meditating together *or* possibly reciting a heartfelt dedication to one another. Whichever you choose, a spiritual component always enhances the lovemaking experience. Such a connection honors God, as well as the divine within each other. This spiritual component sets the tone for the entire lovemaking experience. It activates the upper chakras, just as the sexual energy activates the lower chakras. **Sharing a prayerful moment is one of the purest ways to bring two lovers together.**

Sensual Accents

An awakened state of sexuality not only activates the body's nervous system but also creates a heightened awareness of the senses. In return, the heightened senses raise the sexual experience to a higher level. Although many spiritual paths tend to ignore or deny the body and its senses, in sacred sexuality, you are encouraged to explore every sensation. **Focusing on a sensation (without becoming consumed) is like a meditation that keeps you in the moment.** Your complete awareness is focused on the here and now.

Enjoy every sense and sensation. Use each sensation as a point of focused awareness, as in meditation. Then bask in each sensation as if nothing else exists. Expanding sensual awareness results in a feeling of liberation from physical limitations. Sense-uality nurtures greater sex-uality, which, in turn, awakens more sensuality, and the cycle continues.

Each of the senses is related to one or more of the chakras in the energy system and also to one or more of the cranial nerves in the skull. As you stimulate one of the senses, you activate the chakras, energy systems, cranial nerves, and cranial fluid.

According to *The Prana Upanishad*, an ancient Hindu text, the body is interconnected by the five elements of *earth, water, fire, air,* and *ether*. Each of these elements is related to one of the five senses of *touch, taste, sight, smell,* and *sound*–respectively. Since sacred sexuality involves raising the level of sensual awareness, it is wise to make use of any tools that appeal to and awaken each of these senses. Once you reach the limit of your five senses, it's possible to expand beyond that limit. So take your partner through at least one of each sense-awakening exercise or technique–in any order. For example, prepare your love chamber by using essential oils to awaken the sense of smell, playing music to awaken the sense of sound, dancing to awaken the sense of sight, feeding your partner sweet fruit to awaken taste, and giving him or her an energy massage for the sense of touch. In combination, these suggestions or rituals have a very arousing affect.

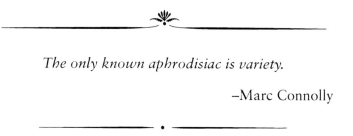

The only known aphrodisiac is variety.

–Marc Connolly

TOUCH (Earth)

- Foods–In addition to its value in the taste category, food provides a wonderful connection between lovers when they feed each other. Fresh fruits are the best, especially topped with whipped cream.
- Bathe Together–Use quality bath oils, bath salts or bubble bath.
- Body Massage–Massage is an excellent way to experience touch. It's healing and can convey love and tenderness. Keep in mind that the lighter the touch, the more sensual the experience.
- Room Temperature–Set a moderate temperature on the thermostat. The room used for lovemaking should be neither too hot nor too cold.
- Genital Awakening Exercises–Use energetic massage techniques and teasing touch to awaken the body through physical sensations.

TASTE (Water)

- Fruit–The most common choices for pleasuring through the sense of taste are cool, fresh, sweet grapes, strawberries, figs and the like. Other succulent choices are peaches, mango, melons or papaya.
- Wine–Some couples often enjoy adding wine to their lovemaking session. But remember, drinking too much can numb the senses, which is counterproductive to sacred sexuality.
- Essential Oils and Massage Oils–Although all scented oils are gifts to the olfactory sense, they can also be delights to the taste buds. There are edible massage oils (from chocolate to cherry) and essential oils (from citrus to lavender).

SIGHT (Fire)

- Clean Environment–Since first impressions often set the tone for experiences, the environment for lovemaking should be pleasing to the eye.
- Candles–Use clean-burning candles with appealing, but not overly perfumed, scents.
- Flowers–Vividly colorful flowers (the more colorful the better) are pleasing to the eyes–the windows to the soul.
- Fruit–Like flowers, colorful fruit, arranged in a basket or on a tray, can emit a subtle aroma, while also being attractive to the eye.

- Dancing–Whether you are partially dressed, totally naked or wearing an eye-pleasing costume, performing an exotic or seductive dance for your partner is a great way to bring playfulness and spontaneity into the lovemaking environment and your relationship.
- Warm Lighting–Rather than shutting off all the lights, allow the glow from candles to illuminate both of you. Be sure you can see into each other's eyes.

SMELL (Air)

- Scented Candles–Use quality candles with a scent that is appealing to you and your lover.
- Flowers–Choose fragrant and exotic flowers whenever possible.
- Fruit–The aroma of fresh fruit and wine is very pleasant to the nose. Play such sensual games as blindfolding, taking turns absorbing the scent of a piece of fruit, and then guessing what it is.
- Water Mister–Mix water and eucalyptus or peppermint oil in a sprayer and lightly mist the room.
- Bath Products–Use quality oils, bath beads or bubble bath.
- Scented Oils–Many pure essential oils are now available. When used with a diffuser, the oil's subtle fragrance will permeate a room without the smoke of burning incense. Using just the right scented massage oil can increase the recipient's desire to be touched.
- Incense–If agreeable to both partners, a small amount of incense can be a treat. Incense should be used in moderation or burned before foreplay, so the smoke has time to clear while the scent lingers.
- Potpourri–When the fragrance of incense or oils is not satisfactory, try a simple, natural potpourri. Use a mixture with citrus and cinnamon, both sensually invigorating.
- Clean Linens–When a bed is used for lovemaking, it's an added sensuous pleasure for lovers to feel the contact of fresh sheets. Knowing that the bed has been specially prepared for this occasion gives added sensual pleasure.
- Deodorant–Some sex educators believe the body should be made to smell as pleasant as possible, while others believe it's better to maintain the body's natural scents. Both opinions have validity. However, there is a difference between body *scent* and body *odor*. Often the scents emitted through the glands and pores of the body are an amazing

aphrodisiac. On the other hand, when toxins or strong smells like garlic leak through the pores, it can be negatively overwhelming and a real turnoff. It also sends unpleasant messages to your lover about your health and self-care.

SOUND (Ether)

- Music–Have music playing in the background to enhance the energy but not loud enough to become a distraction. Most lovers agree that it's best to play music that is not too hard or too soft. Avoid music with excessive lyrics. Of course there are certainly exceptions like the sultry music of *Sade*, *Enigma* or *Enchanted*. Light jazz is another common favorite.
- Nature Sounds–Sounds from nature can be either played on the stereo or experienced as the real thing.
- Poetry–Play tapes of romantic or erotic poetry or recite your own poems to each other. Often times, writing your own erotic stories or poems awakens deeper levels of romance and sexuality.
- Moans–There is probably no sound that is more sexually stimulating than that of your lover's moan (or your own, for that matter). In fact, moaning tends to evoke orgasm.

Awakening the Senses

The following techniques are helpful for awakening the senses. There is one technique offered for each of the senses. For more ideas, consult other books on developing intimacy and sexuality.

TECHNIQUE:
Sensual Contact (Touch)

The first thing to remember about the sense of touch is that your skin is directly related to your brain and is therefore the brain's environmental scout. What the skin perceives, the brain will respond to. When you tease and arouse the skin, the brain sends messages of response throughout the body. The following technique can be done on the entire body or on any selected portion.

STEP 1: Discuss who will *give* and who will *receive* the sensual touch first. Then discuss the depth of contact you each prefer. Keep in mind that with touch, more is *not* always better. In fact, when using touch to arouse the senses, the lighter the touch, the more feeling evoked.

STEP 2: Play soft music and create some soothing aromas. The recipient (or both partners) should now disrobe.

STEP 3: Place a hand over the recipient's heart, while both partners center and pray.

STEP 4: Once contact is made with the love energy of the heart, imagine spreading the energy throughout your partner's heart as you drag or stroke the body with your palms and fingertips.

STEP 5: When this energy is evenly distributed throughout the torso and limbs, draw it towards the genitals with a loving, yet sensually teasing, intent.

STEP 6: After it is clear that the recipient is responding to the movement of sensual energy into his or her genitals, de-tumesce the body and lovingly remind him or her to concentrate on absorbing the energy into the cells of their being. If both partners agree, the excitation can also be turned into passionate lovemaking.

TECHNIQUE:
The Sensual Mouth (Taste)

The following technique is to be done with a partner. If you take time to savor the food and the experience, you may find this technique to be highly erotic. As you entice your partner with a sensual piece of fruit (or whatever food you choose), closely observe his or her body, especially the lips, and sense what is happening. If done properly, this technique is extremely arousing. Add some teasing comments such as, "You *really* want it don't you?" Make your partner long for a bite. As your partner reaches out physically and energetically, it's a sign that their body is coming to life.

STEP 1: Place some of your favorite fruit or desert in a bowl.

STEP 2: Before allowing your partner to deeply absorb the scent and taste of the chosen food, make sure he or she is comfortably lying or seated.

STEP 3: Select an item for your lover to eat. Have them savor it with their nose, then lips, tongue, and mouth.

STEP 4: Ask your lover to take his or her time and focus on each and every sensation arising from the food. Have them slowly suck it, lick it, and rub it around the inside of their mouth before sensually chewing it. Ask your lover to "make love" to the piece of food the way that he or she will make love to you.

TECHNIQUE:

Dancing (Sight)

Dancing is a powerful form of non-verbal communication. Not only can spontaneous dancing or movement shake off physical and energetic tensions, dancing can also seduce your partner and awaken a feeling of playfulness. To build the sensual mood, shift from rhythmic to sensual movements (or vice versa), as you create a dance for his or her eyes only. Dancing for your partner is a great way to honor them with a gift.

STEP 1: Ladies first! Dress lightly with something to entice your lover's imagination.

STEP 2: Play sensuous music loud enough to move your soul into activity.

STEP 3: Use your yin energy to your advantage. Include round, seductive movements with scarves dangling from your fingers, as you dance the dance of Shakti.

STEP 4: As your dance ends, make your way to where you can sit comfortably while your lover brings forth his yang energy.

STEP 5: Now for the male! Dance around the room with passion and vigor, working to get your lover's attention, while increasing sexual energy as you dance the dance of Shiva.

STEP 6: As your dance ends, move toward your lover, sweep her up and invite her to share in a mutual dance of ecstasy. Begin slowly (honoring the yin energy) and progress to more intense movements (honoring the yang energy). Allow this dance to be spontaneous, erotic, and passionate.

STEP 7: When you are done, embrace each other and kiss passionately. Then, let nature take its course.

TECHNIQUE:

Aromatherapy (Smell)

There are many items and products that can bring pleasant aromas into your life and love chamber. These include incense, oils, fresh flowers, and candles. Be sure the fragrance you choose appeals to both you and your lover, since not everyone likes the same scent. Quality is also important, as not all oils are hypo-allergenic. So be careful when applying *pure* oils directly to the skin because some can cause irritation. Use oils that have been diluted, or dilute them by mixing a few drops with another base oil, such as almond oil.

Aromatherapy, in the form of oils or vibrational essences, was used by long-forgotten, ancient civilizations and then adopted by their descendants–the Egyptians, Chinese, Persians, Africans, East Indians, and later, Europeans. Powerful oil combinations were used to anoint the living and the dead. Myrrh was one of the most popular and effective healing oils used by the ancient Egyptians. Myrrh was brought to Jesus both at birth and death.

Oils have also been used as aphrodisiacs since time immemorial–the most popular of these being ylang-ylang. Other common fragrances to enhance a sensual environment include jasmine, clary sage, citrus (such as orange), patchouli, vanilla, rose, and sandalwood. Most of these scents are commonly used for relieving sexual tension, calming the nervous system, evoking deep sensual desire, and awakening the senses. At times, partners may prefer a blend of fragrances, rather than only *one* oil.

STEP 1: Take a moment with your partner to select a few favorite edible oils.

STEP 2: Without revealing where, place a few drops of your partner's favorite oils on different parts of your body.

STEP 3: Blindfold your partner and then lie back. Ask him or her to browse and sniff your entire body to see if they can discern what oils you have placed on which parts of your body.

STEP 4: If your partner can guess which oil is placed on which body part, allow them to lick it off. If your partner misses the spot, ask him or her to move on. You can give them another chance later.

STEP 5: When your partner is finished, switch places and repeat the exercise.

TECHNIQUE:
Poetry and Music (Sound)

Just the *thought* of writing or performing an erotic or romantic poem, short story or song for your lover might be intimidating for some people. After all, there is always a chance your lover might not like it, or worse, he or she might laugh at you. Chances are, though, that they will like it and not laugh. However, confronting such fears is important for your personal development.

Writing a poem or short story will stretch your mind, imagination, and self-confidence. When writing, use an erotic theme and let yourself go. Be loving, yet provocative. Write words that express your deepest desires and blend them with the fantasies of your partner.

Chanting from sacred texts, quoting from epics and dramas, improvising poetry...are great sexual aids.

–Kama Sutra

STEP 1: When you are in a sensual mood, read or watch a movie that evokes arousal.

STEP 2: Then spend time in quiet contemplation or meditation on a sensual feeling or theme. Allow the inspiration for a song or story to come to you. It may come in little pieces, which you can fill in later, or it may come as a whole story. Either way, stay open.

STEP 3: Let the inspiration and writing unfold on its own. Avoid over-analyzing and self-doubt. As you write, do what you can to tune into the collective heart and mind of humanity. Focus on what might arouse your partner and yourself.

STEP 4: You might choose such a theme as walking in the woods or on a beach and meeting a stranger who sweeps you away into lovemaking. You might choose to blend an erotic message to a lover with a love song to God.

STEP 5: When sharing your writing with your partner, be courageous. Assist him or her to get comfortable and offer a drink or light snack.

STEP 6: Leave the room and remove your clothes or change into something sexy.

STEP 7: When you return, ask your partner to relax and take a few deep breaths, as you do the same. Ask him or her to close their eyes, listen,

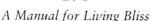
and visualize each detail of what you read or perform.

STEP 8: Begin reading but remember to pace yourself. Read slowly, allowing the pauses to build excitement and anticipation.

STEP 9: When you are finished, your partner will feel aroused as well as appreciative for your creative effort. You can now move on to other forms of awakening the senses, connecting, pleasuring or intercourse.

Love is my ointment, my lubrication, my wetness that wells from deep inside me. Love keeps the body young, the joints oiled. Love is the tingling up the spine, to the neck, into the head. Love is soft. Love is forever. Love is the sunrise and sunset that continue infinitely. Love is the only constant, the indistinguishable. Love is the beginning, and love will be the end. Love is why I am here.

–Valerie Brooks *(Tantric Awakening)*

CHAPTER 10

Cleansing

The Breath

Although most individuals are not conscious of the condition of their own breath, this is certainly something that can "make or break" an intimate moment–even before there is actual contact. Notice how, in the movies, someone who is expecting a date, quickly checks his (or her) breath. Unfortunately, some individuals and cultures aren't very conscientious about such matters. What they fail to realize is that bad breath is not only a "turnoff" but is also a possible sign of poor health or an unclean mouth. One of the best remedies is to thoroughly brush and floss your teeth regularly. It's also wise to use peroxide and mouthwash to clean and disinfect. Even if it feels awkward to discuss bad breath, communication on this matter is essential since honesty is an important part of intimacy.

Grooming

Some Taoist schools teach that a shaved yoni awakens the memory and vitality of youthfulness. Among practitioners of sacred sex, trimming or completely shaving pubic hair is a common practice. A freshly shaved, smooth yoni, for example, can bring added pleasure to both partners during intercourse or oral sex. It permits a warm and sensual, skin-to-skin contact and connection. A shaved yoni is more sensitive during lovemaking or at any other moment of the day. Once it's shaved, the yoni must be *kept* smoothly shaved to prevent stubble burns on a partner's genitals. The shaved or trimmed pubic hair around a *penis* also enhances pleasure. Some men prefer trimming simply because it makes the penis appear larger.

When you shave for the first time, the pubic area may itch for several days. To ease the skin-rash sensation, try using vitamin E lotion or aloe vera as an external soothing ointment. Of course shaving is only one way to remove hair from the yoni (or body). Some women prefer waxing. Whichever the choice, if you decide it's something you'd like to experience, then shave completely and go outside wearing a light, flowing dress but without underwear. Feel the air caressing and teasing your shaved yoni. It's fun to have this little, sensual secret as you walk by others.

Also be sure to keep your hands and fingernails clean and well-groomed. Your nails should not be too long, as they can scratch or cut.

Cleansing the Body

For the sake and safety of cleanliness and good hygiene, make bathing or showering together a major part of foreplay. Such cleansings offer an opportunity to introduce bath gels or essential oils. The resulting scent and feeling of being clean and fresh are wonderful, soothing aphrodisiacs.

Cleaning and preparing the body for lovemaking can be seen as acts of self-love arising from a sense of self-worth. Such care and preparation are also statements about the importance of your lover. The ancients were detailed in their descriptions of how to wash and perfume the body. They considered washing to be symbolic of self-purification—not unlike a baptism. Aside from the symbolism of *cleansing*, washing each other's body provides quality, physical contact. In so doing, lovers become more intimately aware of each other's anatomy. Besides, lightly scented, slippery skin feels wonderful.

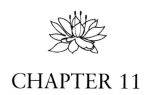

CHAPTER 11

Communicating and Connecting

Clarity of Intent

Communication, especially about rules and intent, is vital for any intimate relationship or encounter. In fact, communication is *so* important that, for partners who are just getting to know each other, it's even more crucial than the usual initial part of foreplay–"setting the environment." Good communication also assists in creating an even better mood and environment. **Clarity of intent is required within *you* before you can share your intentions with friends and selected lovers.**

Setting the Rules of Engagement

Setting "rules of engagement" provides greater safety and responsibility in any relationship but is especially necessary for intimate relations. All partners must have a clear awareness of (and be in agreement with) the intent, rules, and boundaries of a sacred sexual encounter.

If more couples would demonstrate the maturity and responsibility to discuss and agree upon some rules *before* they engage in sexual contact (and stick to these agreements), it would greatly contribute to their emotional health and safety. Instead, couples often rush into a sexual encounter without clarity on the potential outcome. In some cases, the woman gets pregnant, surprises her partner with the news, and is shocked that he wants to abort the baby–or chooses not to be involved in the child's life. Such tragic outcomes need not exist or could be lessened if more lovers would clarify the intent of their relationships, set some rules, and as often as possible stick to their agreements.

Spiritually and psychologically healthy people occasionally enjoy playing with forms of "domination and submission." There are several differences, however, between healthy and unhealthy exploration. **Healthy forms of domination and submission sex-play always exhibit clear boundaries, involve no excessive pain (or worse), and occur between individuals who hold *love* and responsibility as their focus.** Healthy bondage is used only to deepen connection and to playfully learn, explore, and heighten arousal. Within these boundaries, couples are free to explore more erotic forms of sex, such as tying up or spanking each other.

The following are examples of areas where "rules of engagement" should be established. Each person or couple can add or subtract from this list to fit preferences and lifestyles.

1. Whether or not to use birth control.

2. Whether or not to have *any* unprotected genital contact.

3. How far and how fast the experience will go–or the relationship for that matter.

4. What will be done in the event of an accidental pregnancy.

5. Sharing history of STD's.

6. Whether or not it's okay to have an orgasm in your partner's mouth.

7. Where you stand with each other emotionally.

Signal Words and Safety Words

Using "signal words" is a natural extension of establishing rules of engagement. For example, if a couple is sexually active, it's important that they have a means of clearly communicating their likes and dislikes during sex-play. Additionally, "safety words" are necessary, especially for couples who are more experimental or intense with their lovemaking. In such cases, "safety words" are used to signal the presence of a comfort zone beyond which there would be a lack of safety. Safety words also signal when the threshold of comfort has been exceeded, and the sacredness of the encounter is at risk. These signal words should preferably be chosen *before* intimate encounters, but sometimes the need arises *during* the lovemaking experience. Either way, the "signal words" need to be clear–especially if there is a great deal of sexploration.

You may have heard some people jokingly describing their passionate cries as "Don't...stop!" In this example, are they saying, "Don't stop–doing what you are doing"? Or, are they saying, "Please! Don't do what you are doing and STOP immediately"? From this simple example, it becomes clear that words can mean different things to different people under different circumstances.

Couples who play with intense forms of lovemaking are usually clear about the words they use to express when their boundaries of safety and comfort have been crossed. If, for instance, they play with mild or major forms of domination wherein one lover *ties up* the other lover, the one who is tied up might pretend to playfully struggle. The tied lover might even tease the dominating lover by saying, "No! You are not going to have me!" Nevertheless, the dominating lover forces the tied lover into submission and makes love to him or her. But all the while, it's just a game of role-playing. Yet, if being tied up becomes too intense for the receiver, signal words like "Stop!" or "It's too much!" would make the dominating lover back off and release the tied up partner. Thus, prearranged signal words create a feeling of safety, allowing for greater sexual experimentation while maintaining this safety as the foundation of the sexual experience.

Discussing Safe Sex

There are at least two forms of safety that should be considered when discussing "safe sex." The first form involves physical safety and health considerations. The second, involves emotional safety, the importance of which cannot be overstated–especially if a person has any history of sexual trauma.

The need for safe sex and the perilous alternatives have many people paralyzed with fear concerning sexual activity. The issue is worsened by the fact that the so-called "experts" do not seem to agree on the causes and cures of many of the sexually transmittable diseases. However, with a little understanding of STD's, individuals can become empowered to make healthy choices concerning their sexuality.

Generally, the concept of physically safe sex involves the avoidance of exchanging body fluids–unless you are in a monogamous relationship and both partners have tested free of STD's. If you are *not* in such a relationship, then it's best to either abstain from sex altogether or have sensual contact without fluid exchange. Since these choices are not preferable to most individuals, the best way to avoid contracting or transferring STD's (including the HIV virus) when having full contact is to use oral protection or a condom–preferably coated with spermicide containing Nonoxynol-9.

Some of the most common (but not fatal) STD's include the following:

- CHLAMYDIA–a contagious bacterial infection that is easily cleared up with medication.
- GENITAL WARTS–a contagious viral infection that appears as warts in the genital region. It can be managed effectively with medicine, but medical science has no known cure.
- GENITAL HERPES–is a contagious viral infection that appears as painful blisters in the genital region. It can be managed effectively with medicine, but medical science has no known cure.
- HEPATITIS B and HEPATITIS C are two different viruses that (in a small percentage of people) can be sexually transmitted and create long term, recurrent liver disease. Hepatitis C *can* be fatal over time, but many individuals continue to survive for long periods.

Communicating Your Needs

Communicating your needs is different from using signal words for safety. Communicating your needs involves recognizing the importance of an ongoing dialog to maintain the clarity, integrity, and boundaries that define what you want from the experience. Communicating needs also involves more than just telling your partner you really like a certain act he or she performs. **Although, couples *should* verbalize each other's preferences, "turn-ons" and "turn-offs," they should also discuss emotional and spiritual preferences.** Such information helps partners become the best possible lovers. After all, telling your partner is the easiest and surest way for him or her to discover what you want and what you most enjoy.

During lovemaking, there should be constant communication between partners. If you are being pleasured, and a specific touch feels good, let your partner know. The same applies for something that does not feel good. When learning to pleasure your partner, ask plenty of questions about his or her likes and dislikes, preferences and boundaries. Your partner can respond with physical movements, verbal replies or moans.

When I am...able to share what I am truly feeling, my entire body and breath come alive. My body responds to my courage and the truth, it vibrates, it pulsates, it trembles. This makes me...realize that I am not really being vulnerable to another but rather to myself.

–Diana Richardson *(The Heart of Tantric Sex)*

Using Communication to Maintain and Increase Arousal

Communicating to maintain or increase arousal is a natural progression from communicating needs. It involves using dialog to turn each other on and to stay turned on. However, communication also goes beyond dialog. It includes using sounds, such as moans, to express what feels good and what you want more of. You can use erotic dialog to arouse your lover. It turns them on and breaks down his or her resistance and inhibitions. Also, telling your lover that you are aware of what he or she wants and how badly they want it allows your lover to feel and crave it more deeply.

The more you communicate with the partner you are pleasuring, the more willing he or she will be to surrender. You earn your partner's trust partly through your confidence, skill, attention, creativity, and clear intent.

It's up to you to get what you want from your lover. Other than communicating needs, the person being pleasured should do very little–except for relaxing and letting go. Although communication skills come into play even before you make physical contact, their importance continues throughout an encounter–until, of course, the two partners no longer need words to communicate. Up to that point, each partner should personally demonstrate to the other how and where he or she would like to be touched, with how much pressure, and for how long.

Learning to sense when to add stimulation and when to back off makes you a better lover *and* a better person. This level of sensitivity means connecting with your lover at levels you may have never known. You *may* think you are two bodies simply having sex (the biological equivalent to nerve stimulation), but in reality, you are two souls connecting (the spiritual equivalent of returning to Eden).

When communicating, be sure to let your partner know how well he or she is doing. You can also tactfully ask them to alter or fine-tune what he or she is doing. Let your partner know if these alterations increase arousal. Also be sure to continue giving acknowledgment throughout intimate contact and sexual experiences. That way, your partner knows exactly how he or she is doing and how you are feeling. Acknowledgement or feedback not only acts as a turn on and makes both partners feel better, it keeps both of them present and focused.

Sexually arouse your lover by telling him or her what you intend to do to his or her genitals. In so doing, you bring *their* attention to it, as well as your own. Tell your lover that you can feel him or her wanting more and that you're going to bring satisfaction if he or she will show you how badly they want it. This interaction will turn on both of you, while opening up a deeper level of communication. As your lover *asks* for more, they open up to *feeling* more.

Point out, or acknowledge, to your partner, every time you hear a moan or when you feel subtle things like heat or moisture coming from his or her genitals. Again, let them know when you are going to do something to his or her sexual organs and tease him or her with a description of what you will do. This mental teasing causes your partner's consciousness (followed by energy) to flow to the region being discussed. When you touch any part of your lover's body (particularly the sexual organs), tell him or her how good it feels and why. Describe how soft their skin or pubic hair feels, especially if clean-shaven.

There are two ways to become synchronized with your partner: by learning to recognize signs of pleasure in your partner *and* by asking what he or she would like you to do to intensify that pleasure. **The more you focus on the pleasure of your partner, the greater will be your ability to expand and intensify that pleasure.**

Fantasy, which involves the use of imagination, is also crucial for enhancing any sexual experience. First of all, imagination can be used to increase your presence and connection to the moment, such as when you use your lover's fantasies to increase arousal. Secondly, since imagination is a heart-centered faculty, when using this creative level of consciousness, you and your lover are also sharing your hearts. On the other hand, indulging in fantasies that take you away from the present moment (or from your lover) is a misuse of the tool of imagination, especially in sacred sexuality.

Breathing and Toning: The Two Become One

"And the two shall be one" is one of the oldest and most common descriptions of a sacred relationship. This phrase is often mistakenly thought to mean that two individual halves merge to become one whole, complete person. However, it actually means that two people will share the commitment to discover *their own* personal completeness, after which they can choose to share their wholeness with each other. There are numerous exercises that can enhance and facilitate this sense of joining as one.

Some partners find that adding a sound such as toning to some of the breathing exercises takes the process to a whole new level of mutual connectedness. If you choose to experiment with toning, do not attempt to "sing" a musical note, nor should you think of this as chanting "Ohmmm." With toning there is no specific sound. Begin by taking a deep breath, and then on your exhale simply hum a sound. But try to match sounds between you and your partner. As your mouths slowly open, you will discover that the hum gradually grows louder and expands into an "oooouuuu" (which sounds like "you"). Eventually, as you match each other, the sound begins to reverberate back and forth between the two of you, creating a sense of oneness. Toning was used by ancient civilizations to break up old, crystallized cellular patterns and thought-forms.

There are two primary styles of breathing for a couple to share–these are "synchronized breathing" and "alternate breathing." With *synchronized breathing*, or breathing in sync with your partner, you both inhale and exhale at the same time. This type of breathing is intended to increase connection, rather than arousal. Synchronized breathing is also an effective tool for facilitating the transfer of energy from one partner to the other.

With *alternate breathing*, one partner inhales as the other exhales and vice versa. As with synchronized breathing, this breathing is beneficial when added to exercises that include the transfer of energy from one partner to the other.

There comes a moment when more intimate sexual contact occurs with an extraordinary mutuality.

–Alan Watts

TECHNIQUE:
Connecting Third Eye

The third eye is traditionally revered as the energy center of clairvoyance (clear-sightedness) or psychic abilities. By joining with another soul and mutually sharing the energy of your third eye, you can awaken spiritual vision between you and your partner and transcend human perceptions.

STEP 1: Decide who will be the sender and who the receiver. Then lie down on your sides facing each other with your feet at far ends away from each other.

STEP 2: Touch foreheads.

STEP 3: Begin breathing together. Either synchronize your breathing (in and out at the same time) or alternate your breathing (one partner inhales as the other exhales).

STEP4:While remaining present and breathing together, hold the intention of exchanging energy through your third eye for approximately three minutes. This intent should be gentle and subtle, since energy sent into the third eye can be overwhelming.

STEP 5: When both partners are ready, have the sender extend loving thoughts and feelings to the mind of the receiver, who passively absorbs these messages. Then switch roles.

STEP 6: After both partners have sent and received loving energy, let all thoughts and feelings dissolve, except for the feeling and vision of being united as one body and soul with no separation between you.

CHAPTER 12

Kissing and Mouthplay

Kissing Breath

Before your mouth ever makes contact with your lover's, your breath can be conveying messages of desire and sensuality. Each in-breath can be a method of drawing in the essence of your lover. Similar to how your eyes widen when you see something wonderful or you inhale deeply when you smell something pleasant, your in-breath suggests you can "taste" your lover from several inches away. Your out-breath sends a message to your lover that you are on the way and getting closer by the second. In practice, this might feel as though you are lightly sucking in air and gently blowing it out. Breathing in and out in this sensuous fashion, while focusing on your lover's response, will arouse wonderful sensations. You can choose to play with the less responsive areas of the body to evoke a greater awareness there, or you can target the obviously pleasurable areas and drive your lover wild.

Biting

Biting can be done on nearly every part of the external anatomy, with the amount of pressure varying from the lightest nip to the firmest (but never hard) grip. Biting is one of many ways to awaken sensations of a specific region or throughout the entire body.

In the *Kama Sutra*, biting is considered such a crucial part of lovemaking that several variations are noted (as with kissing and intercourse). These variations are as follows:

1. The Hidden Bite–leaves redness but no other mark.

2. The Pointed Bite–uses only the two upper and two lower teeth.

3. The Line of Jewels–uses as many teeth as possible in a big bite.

4. The Line of Jewels Point–uses as many teeth as possible in a small bite.

5. The Coral (lips) and Jewel (teeth) Bite–uses lips *and* teeth to grab hold.

Licking

Before lovers indulge in the art of tongue-play on the body, they should make sure the body and mouth are clean. To reduce the chance of spreading germs, it's wise to clean the mouth by brushing the teeth, flossing, and gargling with an antiseptic mouthwash.

When indulging in tongue-play, remember these basic guidelines. First, always work in the direction of the genitals. Second, choose intuitively where to lick. Avoid being methodical or spending too much time licking your partner's body. Third, consciously and lovingly tease your partner as you lick him or her. The licking should be enticing and stimulating, making them want more; but don't "give in" too quickly. Instead, take your time and find the right pace. Fourth, feel free to add in some spontaneous sucks and bites. Finally, remember to have a refreshing drink nearby to keep your tongue moist.

Primary Types of Mouth Kisses

From the time of infancy, we use our mouths to help us explore the world. As adults, we can connect more deeply with our lovers by use of the mouth, lips, and tongue. This deep connection is like a mystical experience, since it involves a shift of awareness from the self (kissing or being kissed) to an ecstatic experience triggered by melding with our lovers' energy, or essence. We reach this state by letting go and surrendering to the experience of kissing, while simultaneously holding the intent of sharing love.

Most people consider the lips to be an erogenous zone that is *responsive* as well as capable of *evoking* a response. In the art of face reading, the lips are seen as symbolizing the genital region of the body. The upper lip is considered by Tantrists to be a special erogenous zone for a woman, since it has an invisible channel, or meridian, linking it directly to the clitoris. Notice how common it is for advertisers to use the image of a woman licking her upper lip and how seductive this image appears. The same is true for the lower lip of a man.

Kissing is a highly sensual experience for the body and soul. The forms and styles of kissing range from a simple, quick peck on the lips or cheek to the deepest passionate exchange. Tantric masters refer to kissing as the *"meeting of the upper gates."* Contact between the genitals is the *"meeting of the lower gates."* These "gates" designate the opening where an inward and outward exchange, or transfer, of energy takes place.

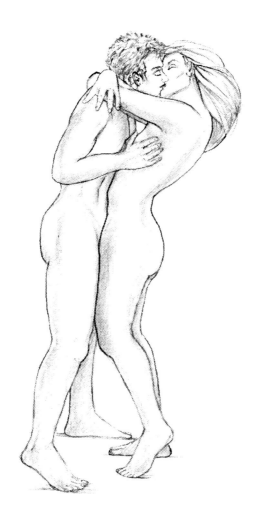

The passionate kiss

When kissing your lover's mouth, be playful and explore. Kiss each lip separately; kiss gently and lovingly and then intensely and passionately; kiss for a few seconds and for twenty minutes; kiss with eyes open and closed.

There are three primary types of kisses:

1. The Minimal Kiss–Two people making quick contact with their mouths.
2. The Sensual Kiss–The mouths make longer contact, the lips give, and the heads tilt.
3. The Passionate Kiss–The mouths are open. The tongues are used, and the bodies respond.

TECHNIQUE:

Deepening Your Kiss

For some individuals, kissing is as intimate as intercourse, which makes sense considering the mouths are reflexes of the genitals. Many prostitutes are willing to share their bodies through oral sex and intercourse, yet prefer to avoid kissing their clients. To connect with our mouths means our eyes may meet as well–adding another level of intimacy. Incidentally, you do not have to *be* in love to *kiss* with love.

STEP 1: Take a few minutes to connect with your partner. Breathe together and exchange loving compliments.

STEP 2: Join mouths with your partner. Match your lip movements, and then move from a minimal kiss to a sensual kiss, wherein the lips soften but do not completely open.

STEP 3: Slide your mouths slightly to where the man has the woman's upper lip in his mouth and the woman has the man's lower lip in her mouth.

STEP 4: As you suck and lick each other's lip, imagine an energy meridian running from your lip that is being sucked, down to your genitals and stimulating this region.

STEP 5: Once you feel a response in the genitals, allow your mouths to open into a passionate kiss. Move together at a similar pace and with matching movements. Gradually begin to deepen the kiss, but keep it slow. Avoid the temptation to shift into the "heights" of fast kissing. This is fine if agreed upon, but the main goal is to kiss with slow, loving intent. Also avoid kissing with a hard or pointed tongue.

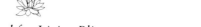
STEP 6: Now focus on the juices in your mouth. Be aware of exchanging your frothy saliva.

STEP 7: Be aware of the loving hold you should have on your partner and tune-in to your hands. Can you kiss your partner at the same time that your hands convey how much you care about him or her?

STEP 8: When your kissing exchange is complete, gently move your lips apart, and soak up the experience as you continue to embrace.

CHAPTER 13

Massaging and Caressing

Touching

It is believed that the brain is the most sensitive erogenous zone mainly because this is where we receive pleasure signals. Yet the skin is a companion to the brain in the developmental stages of a fetus. It is also a sensitive erogenous zone because the skin is the message gatherer for the brain. The body is completely covered by the sensitive skin that has millions of sensors capable of sending whispers of pleasure to the brain. Therefore, the entire body is an erogenous zone that is highly responsive to touch.

When a person yearns to be touched, it surfaces in the body as something called tumescence. Tumescence awakens slight pulsing contractions of muscles in the body and awakens the various endocrine glands.

The ancient practitioners of sacred sexuality taught five *forms* of physical touch: stroking, pinching, scratching, tapping, and squeezing. Each of these can vary in combination, speed, and pressure. Also, in the art or practice of sacred sexuality, there are three *levels,* or depths, of touching and contact:

1. Massaging touch–contacts the body's tissues at various depths.
2. Internal touch–penetrates a body with the fingers, hands, tongue, and penis.
3. Energetic touch–has no *physical* contact with the body, but still evokes a response.

Playful Sexual Exams

Exchanging sexual exams with your partner is a wonderful way to learn, while simultaneously developing greater mutual trust and connection. The sexual exam is like an adult version of "playing doctor." Each partner takes time to examine and explore the other. If you try this exam, be sure to follow a sequence that has a natural flow–such as moving from head to toe or from extremities to genitals. Some tools of the playful exam include a hairbrush, latex gloves, and lubricant. During the exam, you will also use your hands, fingers, tongue, and hair to playfully examine the sensitivity levels of specific areas of your partner's body. Here are some suggestions for the exam:

1. On a male, you can use a hairbrush to trace the pubic hair-growth patterns.
2. Check nipple sensitivity and arousal response by licking and blowing.
3. Trace the lips with one or two fingertips to test the mouth's sensitivity.
4. Rub around the perineum area to test its response.
5. Lick and blow across the genitals to test arousal.
6. Playfully explore the anus by testing your partners response to light stimulation.
7. Take a peek inside the urethra (the hole you urinate from). It should look pink or slightly red in color.

Scratching and Clawing

Scratching, as a form of sex-play, involves using fingernails to grab, claw, or scratch your lover. For some ancient cultures, claw marks were signs that identified you as someone's sexual "territory." Of course, in these modern times, clawing and scratching need not bare the intent of possessiveness that it once did. But, mild demonstrations of clawing and scratching *can* evoke very strong sexual responses in some people. Since light scratching creates tingles in the body and draws greater circulation to the surface of the skin, it also enhances sexual arousal. Lovers might enjoy firmly gripping their partner's butt with their claws, which can also evoke deep arousal. Sometimes lovers can get a little extra passionate and claw firmly enough to slightly break the skin. This can actually be a very erotic experience for some, but pushes the barriers of comfort for others. For lovers who prefer more than just *mild* clawing and scratching, keep in mind that *sacred* sexuality maintains a boundary of love and safety.

Sex Toys

Sex toys have been used throughout the ages. They are not new. Carvings, drawings, and writings from numerous ancient cultures depict women masturbating with stone or wooden phallic objects–now known as dildos.

Today one of the most common sex toys for women is a vibrator. These come in various shapes and sizes from the most simple finger appliance to complex, multi purpose stimulators. Such objects can be a playful part of sexploration. However, since the goal of sacred sexuality is to nurture a greater connection between individuals and Spirit, everything about a sacred sexual encounter must be love-based, or it's not sacred. Any addiction or dependence on such objects as sex toys could stand in the way of this spiritual goal. If such is the case, they should be avoided or used only sparingly. A vibrator should not be used as a replacement for lovemaking, but as a means of awakening the sensual body.

"Ben wa" balls are one of the better toys or tools for awakening the yoni. When placed in the yoni for a few hours, ben wa balls mildly stimulate the inner muscles and nerves of the yoni. They also stimulate sexual secretions, which are good for a woman's overall health.

Sex toys generally fall into one of the following classifications.

1. **Oral Toys**–such as edible oils.
2. **Tactile (skin stimulating) Toys**–such as feathers and scarves.
3. **S & M Toys**–such as whips, leashes, collars, and restraints.
4. **Intercourse Toys**–such as vibrators and various forms of dildos.

Lubricants

Lubricants, as the name implies, are used for their lubricating abilities during manual pleasuring or intercourse. The primary goal of a lubricant is to create smooth contact and prevent irritation to the skin. Lubricants are also chosen for their flavored, edible qualities.

Lubricants, however, are not all created equal. **There are essentially four common types of lubricants:** *water-based, silicone-based, oil-based,* **and** *petroleum-based.* The first two (water or silicone-based) are safe to use with condoms and other rubber products. The latter two (oil or petroleum-based) are not safe with rubber products. Of course, some people prefer to use saliva. But saliva can spread viral or bacterial infections–especially in women who are prone to urinary tract and genital infections. Each type of lubricant has benefits, as well as potential drawbacks. Experiment and discover what works best for you. You can also do further research on the internet or ask your doctor for additional information.

Before choosing a lubricant, first decide whether or not you will be using any rubber products (such as gloves, condoms, and diaphragms). If so, avoid oil and petroleum-based lubricants, as they will break down the rubber, rendering it unsafe as protection. Also, when using any form of lubricant, first pour it on your hands and rub it until it's warm. Then apply it a little at a time to your partner's genitals.

Water-based lubricants are fun to apply; they won't stain the sheets; they are easily washed from the skin; they can be used with latex condoms; and they are often flavored for better taste. The major drawback is that water-based products tend to dry up quickly or become sticky. Therefore it's necessary to keep reapplying–especially if the application is used for long durations. The water-based lubrications on the market vary, but the most well-known are K-Y Jelly and Astroglide. Another thicker lubricant is known by two names–"Sex Grease" for the male and "Sensura" for the female. If you prefer flavored lubricants, try l-D Juicy Lube, as it comes in a variety of flavors.

Water-soluble lubricants are wonderful for lubricating a penis as they spread easier than petroleum products; but again, they dry up quickly. When applying a lubricant to the penis, be sure to include the testicles first.

Then proceed with long strokes from the base to the tip of the penis. The head of the penis (like the clitoris of a woman) should be lubricated last.

A few of the water-soluble lubricants come with the spermicide nonoxynol-9, which has been proven to destroy some STD viruses. But used over an extended period, nonoxynol-9 can cause irritation of the skin, resulting in a burning or stinging sensation to the genitals.

Silicone-based lubricants are, in most respects, similar to water-based lubricants. Yet they retain their lubricating properties longer than water-based lubricants. So a little goes a long way. Like water-based lubricants, silicone will not harm latex, as will oil or petroleum-based lubricants. Yet they can harm sex toys that are made of silicone. So do not mix the two. Silicone-based lubricants are completely waterproof, making them ideal for underwater use.

Oil-based lubricants are usually made from natural products, such as vegetable oils (olive or corn) and nut oils (peanut). Oil-based lubricants, like petroleum-based lubricants, tend to stain fabrics and can be difficult to wash off but are safer to use inside the vagina. Oil-based lubricants destroy latex, so they should never be used with condoms or other rubber materials. Otherwise, oil-based lubricants are good for intercourse, anal sex, and genital pleasuring. Most oil-based lubricants are available in supermarkets, making them easier to find than the fancier lubricants found only in sex shops.

Petroleum-based lubricants are great, in that each application lasts much longer than water-based lubricants, making them easier on the skin. The drawbacks are that, unlike water-based lubricants, petroleum-based jells break down the latex in gloves or condoms; they stain fabrics; they are very difficult to wash off; and of course, they don't taste very good. Petroleum-based lubricants include Vaseline products and baby oil. However, the extra thickness of petroleum-based lubricants makes them a perfect choice to use when massaging the clitoris, which tends to be hypersensitive to direct touch.

Petroleum jelly works best on the clitoris for most women–unless you plan on having intercourse afterwards with the use of a condom. Apply petroleum jelly to the clitoris and begin pleasuring the clitoris by spreading the lubricant around the clitoral hood, which often produces a better response than touching the clitoris directly. Gradually progress to experimenting with direct clitoral pleasuring but keep in mind that direct contact is best only if your partner prefers it.

Sensual Massage

There are several forms of intimate, sensual massage that can create incredible pleasure for lovers. In general, the best way to give a sensual, arousing massage is to rub or tickle the body in the direction of the genitals. When massaging, energizing, or licking your lover, give added attention to the curve of the back (especially on a woman). Stimulating this region can, in itself, arouse the genitals and lubricate the yoni.

Sensual massage is not meant to have the same affects on the body as a deep body massage. **A sensual massage focuses on making connection, creating trust, and stimulating a greater sense of sexual anticipation between lovers.**

When you come to be sensibly touched, the scales will fall from your eyes; and by the penetrating eyes of love you will discern that which your other eyes will never see.

–Francois Fenelon

When giving a sensual massage, remain aware of any subtle shifts that take place in either you or your partner. Be sure to encourage feedback. Additionally, instead of using only hands for massaging, try using your forearms as well. To add playfulness and stimulation, try using blindfolds and use more than just hands to massage your partner. Use your breasts, hair, and genitals, along with provocative dialog.

If you use oil when massaging, be sure to use towels to protect sheets and bed covers. Always warm the oils in your hands or in hot water before applying to your partner's skin. Be sure to use enough so the fingers slide easily, but not so much that it causes your hands to slip off of your lover. Since massage oils are relatively inexpensive, some couples like to use large quantities of oil to create a sensual slide-affect.

To mix oils at home, add a dozen drops of your favorite essential oil to a few ounces of unscented base oil. Either olive or almond oil is a good choice for a base oil because it is healthy for the skin and safe if ingested. You can apply the oil to your partner by rubbing against him or her with *your* lubed-up body. Just the feel of the warm oil is soothing and arousing.

Touching and massaging are a very intimate expression. If the touch feels right, it can set the stage for a wonderful sexual experience. On the other hand, **an insensitive touch can cause physical and psychological tension, which is counterproductive to any sacred sexual encounter.** In general, you are safe to let your feelings be your guide. Make sure that you communicate with your partner and keep close observation of his or her responses.

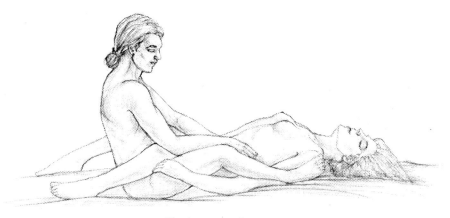

Sharing sensual massage

Other tips to ensure a sensuous, satisfying massage experience include the following:

1. The longer and more subtle the stroke, the more erotic and stimulating the sensation. On the other hand, the deeper, shorter strokes tend to sedate and calm.
2. Take your time.
3. Take turns in the active *and* passive role.
4. Arouse the whole body before reaching for the genitals.
5. After building arousal (tumescence) by stimulating the primary erogenous zones, use the less excitable parts of the body to bring your partner back down (de-tumescence).

There are numerous ways to stimulate the flow of blood and energy to specific body parts, especially the genitals. Here are some suggestions.

1. Gentle Hair Pulling (for men or women): Gently, but firmly, pull the pubic hair, not to cause pain or discomfort but to evoke stimulation of

the pubic region. Pulling the hair causes blood to rush to this region with excitement, creating a prickly sensation in the sex organs.

2. Labia Wiggling (for women): Starting with one side of the outer labia, pinch the labia gently between your thumb and first finger. Gently pull on the labia and shake it rhythmically. Then, proceed to the other lip.

TECHNIQUE:
Sensual Massage Using Your Body

One of the most sensual ways to massage your lover's body is to use your own body. The more skin-to-skin contact the better. With this constant contact, as the oil warms up, so do your bodies. It's wonderful to play some sensual, relaxing music and slither all over your lover.

STEP 1: The partner giving the massage (the active partner) thoroughly lubricates the front of his or her own body. The partner receiving the massage (the passive partner) lies on his (or her) back on top of several towels or expendable sheets.

STEP 2: The active partner lies (chest to chest) on the passive partner with full body contact.

STEP 3: The active partner now sensually rubs his whole body along the surface of the passive partner's body until they are both thoroughly covered with oil.

STEP 4: The active partner occasionally moves his or her pelvis in provocative, grinding motions.

STEP 5: Since you are now both lubed up, switch roles and let the passive partner do the slithering.

STEP 6: If you used *edible* oils, you can now take turns licking the oils off each other's bodies.

Energetic Massage

Energy massaging is different from other forms of massage. Unlike a more traditional massage, there is little or no contact with the skin. Instead, the person giving the massage works with the *energy* emitted from the body of the person receiving, to awaken the energy systems of the person receiving the energy-work.

Energy massage is usually done with bare hands, but some additional tools provide a playful touch. The most common tools used in such a massage are feathers, silk scarves, fur, and velvet. An energy massage can also be combined with the use of aromatic fragrances or food to further entice and excite your lover.

The purpose of an energy massage is to arouse and entice your partner into *wanting* more of you and what you are offering. This is accomplished through a combination of intent, energy movement, hand placement, and sensual dialog–your personal tools of seduction.

In one effective form of energy massage, the man lies back with the woman either sitting between his legs or at his side. Using concentration, visualization, and the energy emitting from her hands and fingers, the woman stimulates and entices her partner's penis–without actually touching him. With no physical contact, she arouses his penis and causes it to move from side to side. This type of massage stimulates an energy exchange between partners, while evoking a growing desire within the male. Provocative dialog will further increase the effectiveness of her energy-work. The purpose of this exercise is not to increasingly frustrate the male, but to tease him in a fashion that builds sexual energy. Once the woman feels she has aroused her partner sufficiently, they can exchange roles. The man can now perform the same exercise on the woman, teasing her yoni and clitoris. Or they might decide to wait until another time for her to receive and, instead, move on to other forms of pleasuring.

Again, teasing between lovers through energy-building is meant to create a closer connection between them, not to create frustration. So it's essential that each partner develops the intuition and instinct to know when to *tease* and when to *ease*.

TECHNIQUE:
Sensing Chakras and Body Temperatures

The greater the sensitivity, the better the lover. Therefore, it's wise to practice exercises and techniques that enhance your ability to see and feel things beyond the dense, material world and body. The following technique encourages you to feel the more subtle aspects of your partner's body, such as the aura, body temperature, and energy emitted from the chakras.

STEP 1: The woman lies back, closes her eyes, practices deep breathing, and relaxes. Her partner sits at her side and does some centering and prayer.

STEP 2: When both partners have become relaxed and centered, the man slowly runs his hands slightly above and across all parts of the woman's body (without making physical contact). The pace should be slow enough for him to remain sensitive to any variations in body temperature from one part of her body to another. He might also sense that some areas create more tingling in his hands than others, especially when he passes over primary energy centers (chakras).

STEP 3: At the same time, the woman tunes in to see if she senses where her partner's hands are at any given time. She tells him where she feels any unique sensations, and he confirms whether or not his hands are in that region.

STEP 4: After the energy scan is completed on the front of her body, the woman turns over for her partner to practice the same exercise on the back of her body.

STEP 5: When this exercise is completed, the man and woman change positions, and he receives while she passes her hands over his body.

Playing The Erogenous Zones

There is a direct, significantly strong relationship between the body's erogenous zones and various other parts of the body. The theory that major organs and glands are reflected (as reflexes) onto the feet, hands, and face is well known to acupuncturists, reflexologists, and face readers. This theory holds especially true for the face. For example, in "face reading," the mouth symbolizes the sexual organs. The face and the sexual center are also connected through what are known as "ring muscles." When one of these ring muscles is stimulated (such as the mouth), another often responds as well (such as the perineum or genitals). Therefore, stimulating the face (especially the mouth) can be very erotic and results in stimulation to the sexual organs.

Although the body is filled with reflex points, some of the most potent points are the sexual organs themselves. There are vital reflexes for major organs and glands along the penis and within the vagina. **When the sexual organs of two lovers unite, a powerful stimulation of healing energy is experienced throughout the whole body.** Consequently, the physical compatibility of partners (in terms of the size and proportion of the sexual organs themselves) takes on a whole new meaning. In this sense a "perfect fit" means the greatest amount of contact between the organs.

Other parts of the body, besides the genitals, also trigger a sexual response. For example, the middle finger of a man doubles as a penis and is related to the man's heart and his sex meridian. The pinkie finger of a woman, however, doubles as the woman's clitoris, as well as her emotions.

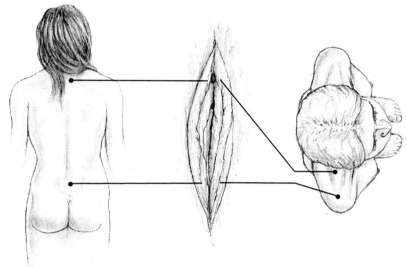

Reflexes of the yoni onto the back and each shoulder

Besides the importance of a specific finger in relation to sexual responses, the hands themselves are very sensitive to kissing, licking, sucking, and massaging. Stimulating the hands sends a powerful wave of sexual energy throughout the whole body–partly due to the hands having reflexes for the whole body.

Even the muscle groups of the body have reflections of the genitals. The yoni, for example, is reflected onto the back muscles of a woman, as well as the top of her shoulders and numerous other body segments. The mouth reflects the vaginal opening and the throat, the vaginal canal. If the mouth is a reflex projection of the yoni the ears would be reflexes for the ovaries. Then, if you turn the anatomy of a woman upside down, her mouth is once again a reflection of her vagina. Her collar bones reflect her pelvic muscles, and her "clitoral legs" are symbolically reflected onto her collar bones. Therefore, the proper contact with this region can sexually arouse a woman.

For a male, nearly all the same reflexes apply. For example, his ears reflect his testicles. The tension that a man habitually carries in his body can make it difficult to access his sexual reflexes. However, releasing the tension in his legs can evoke a sensual response in his penis. His leg muscles might be quite resistant, but it can be done. The trick is to discover if he needs a firm or subtle approach to these muscles.

Learning to Relax, Receive and Surrender

Although it may be "*better* to give than to receive," the truth is that for many of us, it's simply *easier* to give than receive. So we find ourselves busy with giving and rarely taking time to receive. This is because when we're giving (by our choice), we are also still in control. To truly receive means to let go, be vulnerable, seemingly under the loving control of another person, which is a foreign concept for some of us. Nevertheless, there are times when we need to *stop doing* and *just receive*–stop "efforting" and just relax. **Learning to receive is a powerful means of healing issues of unworthiness.** We usually experience love most fully when it's offered by someone we trust. When receiving nurturance from our partners, we experience shades of Love Divine.

To receive a greater amount of pleasure during sensual experiences, relax and *do as little as possible*. Imagine that! You are being told that to receive one of life's greatest pleasures, you need *do nothing*. Yet, ironically, doing nothing is not easy for most people. The act of relaxing and receiving may be hard if you have been conditioned to "take care" of others or if you are distracted by a goal of orgasm.

As soon as you establish a goal during lovemaking, you tense in anticipation and from an attempt to reach that goal. This inevitable tensing might still allow for a peak orgasm, but it lessens the ability to experience a valley or total-being orgasm that relies on a state of relaxing and letting go. This deeper level of orgasm is also contingent upon the awareness that you *are* the bliss and orgasm you seek–there is nowhere to go and nothing to anticipate. So drop all forms of tensing and chasing. **Ecstatic beingness is here, in the now. If it is something you need to achieve, it's in the future; and the future, by definition, is never here now.** You cannot *force* relaxation any more than you can *force* love. But you *can* drop the obstacles of fear and tension that interfere with love and letting go.

Believe it or not, it takes energy to tense any body part. This expending of energy distracts you from feeling the sensations of the moment. Furthermore, tension can restrict the flow of blood and oxygen to the nerves and muscles of the genital area, limiting your ability to feel pleasure and sensual responses.

The following are some guidelines for letting go of tensions:

1. Use *physical* relaxation techniques such as stretching and deep breathing.
2. Evoke greater *emotional* trust through communication and vulnerability.
3. Maintain the mental focus and discipline necessary to gently command each anxious thought and tense muscle to relax and let go.
4. Develop an attitude of *spiritual* surrender to God–something greater than you or your partner.

If you desire an ecstatic experience, remember that the more you relax, the more you can feel. **As you deepen your level of relaxation, you will also increase your ability to absorb the sexual energy deeply into the cells of your body.** Relaxing, in this context, does not imply becoming sleepy or lazy, but rather peaceful, calm, tension-free, and invigorated. Achieving this level of relaxation is difficult if you are busy or too distracted with intense movements or fatigue and physical discomforts.

Once again, **your chances of receiving the greatest amount of pleasure during a sexual experience are increased proportionately to your degree of relaxation.** To increase your level of relaxation, lie still, exerting as little energy as possible, and support your body (particularly the neck, back, and legs) with pillows. As the recipient of pleasure, you will experience various levels of sexual ecstasy when you are relaxed and focusing all your attention on any immediate sensations. Therefore, focus your attention on what you are feeling (physically, energetically, and emotionally) and communicate these feelings to your partner.

Manually Pleasuring Others

This section describes techniques for stimulating men and women to the point of orgasm or even multiple orgasms. It cannot be overemphasized that for most individuals (but not all) achieving orgasms, especially multiple orgasms, involves a process that takes time and is often not accomplished during the first few attempts. **The inability to reach multiple orgasms without months or years of learning and healing does not mean**

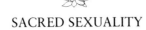

an individual is less sexual or passionate than the person for whom that process is easier. More time and persistence may be needed for some individuals because of genetics, anatomical and physiological variations, personal inhibitions, or physical and emotional traumas.

It's not just giving that brings pleasure; it's also receiving. In concert, these two essential human acts join in a circle of interaction that expands with use. When the circle is complete, the more you give, the more you get, and vice versa.

–George Leonard

The proper technique for manually pleasuring (masturbating) another involves far more than the quick and heavy-handed practices of the clumsy learning stages that some people never outgrow. This is not to say that manual stimulation must always be in your love chamber or that it must always be given an hour to accomplish. There is certainly something to be said about spontaneous pleasuring or intercourse in the form of a playful "quickie." However, time should also be provided for lengthier sessions, which offer results that a quickie could never match. The most powerful forms of manually pleasuring another person to orgasm require an extended amount of attention on the person with whom you are working. If done well, **hand stimulating another person is an art form in itself.** For example, a woman should touch a penis in a fashion that communicates she has found a "pot of gold." Her touch should demonstrate that the act of stimulating her lover's penis arouses *her* as well. The same principle applies to a man making contact with a woman's yoni. Unfortunately, most often a man touches a woman's yoni with a desire to follow through to intercourse or to prove his sexual skills at stimulating his lover. Instead, he should take his time and attentively touch all sections of his lover's yoni with his hands, conveying the message that each part gives him pleasure.

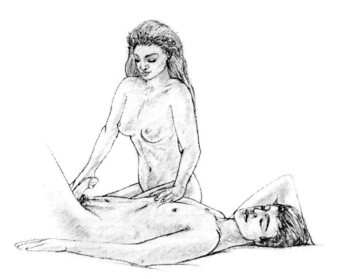

Manually pleasuring others

When pleasuring your partner, be sure you are both as comfortable as possible. There are numerous positions for the giver, but the most common are as follows:

1. *Sitting at the receiver's side* (next to the hip). The giver should have plenty of back support, and the receiver should be comfortable with legs well supported by pillows. Both hands should be free and available to manipulate the genital area.

2. *Sitting in between the receiver's thighs* (facing the genitals). Although this position is similar to the previous one, it is more powerful for the giver and more vulnerable for the receiver. However, because of the angle needed for stimulating the woman's clitoris, a male might prefer the previous position. In either case, both hands of the giver are free for pleasuring.

3. *Lying at the receiver's side* (with head to each other's feet). This position limits the giver to one hand, since the other hand and arm are supporting the upper body. However, with this position that simulates the "69" position, the *giver* is closer to the receiver's genitals.

4. *Sitting over the face of the receiver* (which is easier for the female). The giver sits on the face of the receiver, with each knee placed on the floor or mattress next to each of the receiver's ears and facing in the direction of the receiver's genitals. Once again, one of the giver's hands will be needed to support the weight of the upper body, while the other is used for pleasuring.

Increase the pleasuring experience by learning how to bring your partner up to an ecstatic peak (without cumming) and then down slightly, only to repeat the process again and again. **The best tools for enhancing pleasure are a loving, caring heart, knowledge of proper pleasuring techniques, and intuitive instincts.** Another effective tool for enhancing pleasure involves the ability to alter the sexual experience through conscious intention–the "power of the mind."

A good way to discover the kind of strokes your partner likes is to ask him or her if you may watch them do self-pleasuring so you can learn from what they do. Your partner can also take your hand and guide you through their favorite technique.

Once you tune-in to the energetic flow between you and your partner, you'll be able to alter the intensity of, and responses to, stimulation–seemingly at will. When you are in this zone of heightened awareness, you can use conscious intent to increase the level of arousal. Then, whenever you choose, you can decrease the arousal as well. Again, this kind of connection takes concentration and loving intent. By focusing completely on your partner, you will be able to connect on deeper levels throughout the sexual experience.

When you are finished pleasuring, gradually bring your partner down (known as de-tumescing) with grounding exercises. Let your partner know what you are doing, as you slightly increase the amount of hand pressure and/or by slowing down the strokes. After a few minutes of de-tumescing the pleasuring process, place one hand over your partner's pubic bone (the bone beneath the pubic hair) and press firmly for a few minutes. Then place one hand over your partner's heart center (mid-breastbone) and press firmly. Or do both hand placements simultaneously.

There are times when you will consciously bring your partner completely down. Yet, at other times, you might bring him or her down to a plateau with the intent of coming back up. There are several ways to do this. One way to alter your partner's level of stimulation is to slightly change whatever you are doing–but not too much! Rather than making complete, sudden alterations, make subtle changes from one highly pleasurable form of stimulation to another. But begin slowly. When the time feels right, go back to the original spot of pleasure and take your partner higher.

There are several reasons for bringing your partner down a little: if your partner becomes so excited that his or her breathing becomes too intense, if your partner keeps "leaving their body" and "spacing out," and/or if you want to tease your partner up and down in order to extend their pleasure. However, if it feels like your partner's level of arousal can no longer be increased, you can choose to bring them down gently–like floating in a parachute. In other words, if your partner *does* slip away and their level of arousal decreases with no chance of increasing again, it's important to regain connection and loving control to facilitate their gentle descent. Your partner will appreciate that you are fully present and aware of such subtle shifts in his or her energy levels.

Be sure to *communicate* while you are de-tumescing your partner. With a calming, confident tone, remind your partner to relax. When the pleasuring is concluded, let your partner know how the experience felt to you and ask them to share as well.

In the event that your partner experiences shaking at any time during the pleasuring, reassure them that these spasms are the body's way of processing and channeling the ecstatic, orgasmic energy. In time, most people become accustomed to these surges, and the tremors often relax into deep waves.

IMPORTANT REMINDERS
FOR MANUALLY PLEASURING OTHERS

- Pause to allow the energy that is building to spread through the body.
- Use plenty of lubrication.
- Avoid pressuring your partner or yourself to perform.
- Keep sensually touching your partner's entire body.
- Open your eyes and maintain eye contact whenever possible.
- Remember to be playful, creative, and fun-loving.
- Keep checking to see how your partner is doing.
- Develop a loving, trusting relationship for the best results and responses.
- Make sure your hands and nails are clean and that your nails are very short.

Manually Pleasuring a Woman

Before you begin to manually pleasure your partner, be sure that you have spent time connecting with her–talking, hugging, kissing, and perhaps massaging. It's also essential that she feels safe, desired, and appreciated. Having her legs opened wide feels vulnerable enough, but having someone so close to her genitals might feel excessively awkward. So be attentive and sensitive for any signs of discomfort. **Stay present by keeping your mind focused on what you are doing.** Picture each stroke in your mind. Be sure you acknowledge every pleasurable moan she makes.

TECHNIQUE:

Pleasuring the Clitoris

The clitoris is like a masculine symbol of a woman's sexuality. When excited, it stands at attention like a guard at the kingdom's gate–swelling to as much as twice its original size. An aroused clitoris can be viewed as a woman's way of trying to distract her partner–testing him to see if he is willing to earn his way to her G-spot and, perhaps, on to deeper parts of her soul. Therefore, the clitoris needs to be touched but approached carefully. Most clitoral orgasms occur by stimulation to the clitoris *through* the surrounding hood, rather than directly touching the clitoral head. Think of the art of clitoral stimulation (and all forms of lovemaking) as similar to surfing. You must discover when to press forward and when to back off. There must be no separation between you and the object of your love. Some women enjoy a direct touch, while others need all stimulation to be indirect. Together you must discover what your lover enjoys most.

For women who prefer *direct* stimulation, the best way to stimulate the clitoris is to gently pull the hood back and out of the way. Then place a finger directly on the exposed clitoris. There are several ways to pull back the hood, yet sometimes a woman feels more involved (and aroused) by doing it herself. The most common method is to place the palm of your hand on her pubic mound (just above the clitoris and its hood), press your hand down slightly, and then simultaneously slide her pubic skin upward (towards her navel). This stretches, or pulls, the hood upward and off of the clitoris–thus exposing it.

STEP 1–CREATING A CONNECTION: After foreplay (touching, kissing, and massaging), briefly discuss the intentions of the following exercise with your partner before continuing. Make sure the room is warm to avoid the need for blankets. Place a towel under her in case she releases fluids (ejaculates). Have your partner lie back in a comfortable position with plenty of pillows supporting her body (especially her limbs), so she can completely relax, let go, and surrender. Take a moment to breathe together before you continue with the pleasuring.

Begin to lightly massage and caress your partner's limbs in the direction of her genitals. As you do so, encourage her to breathe deeply. Occasionally remind her to relax, let go, and allow you to pleasure her. Lightly caress her torso–also towards the genitals. Be sure to watch her body language. Eventually, when her pelvis and thighs begin to lift or move, it is an indication that her yoni is ready to be touched.

When pleasuring your partner's extremities, begin with her arms and move to her legs. Try either slow spiral motions or long strokes but always in the direction of her heart or her yoni. For a more sensual effect, stroke her body with only one or two fingers. Otherwise, use all of your fingers or the palm of your hand with light to medium pressure. Pay special attention to the softest parts of the muscles, while continually monitoring her feelings and reactions.

Be sensitive and conscious of each movement as you massage your partner. Remain in the present moment, and let your focus be exclusively on pleasuring her. Be sure to communicate. If you both notice her waves and spasms of orgasmic energy, it's a sign that you are both connected. However, if one of you doesn't notice, it's a sign that one of you is disconnected. It doesn't matter which person may have become disconnected, it's up to you, as facilitator, to reestablish the connection through mental focus, dialog, and contact.

After stroking each arm and leg, move to your partner's breasts. Brush lightly across the nipples, which are probably erect at this point. Then de-tumesce each breast by placing your palm over them and gently but firmly rotating the breasts in circles. You can de-tumesce both breasts at the same time or one at a time. Eventually proceed to her stomach and then pubic region. This entire process of creating a connection should take fifteen to twenty minutes.

After you've completed the energy build up in her limbs and front torso, place your hand gently over her yoni, cupping the whole area (with palm facing towards the yoni). Place your other hand over her heart center. These hand positions maintain the connection between her heart and yoni–love and sexuality.

STEP 2–CONTACTING THE YONI: Apply plenty of oil-based lubricant to your fingers and begin to gently stroke the genitals. Using your fingertips, stroke along the major and minor lips, always in the direction of the clitoris. Eventually, make your way to the clitoris and gently stroke around it without making direct contact. When your partner's body "asks for it," begin to occasionally rub across the clitoris lightly and briefly with a teasing touch.

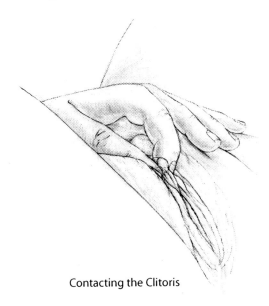

Contacting the Clitoris

STEP 3–STIMULATING THE CLITORIS THROUGH ITS HOOD: Initially rub the clitoris through the surrounding hood of skin. Experiment with various strokes (pressures and directions) to discover what your partner enjoys most. Take the clitoris between your thumb and index finger and gently rub it back and forth in a twisting-like motion. Then switch to another technique. Place the thumb and/or index finger of your free hand behind the upper portion of the clitoris, pinning it in position, while the lubricated index and middle fingers of your other hand begin to gently stimulate the clitoris through the hood.

STEP 4–DIRECTLY STIMULATING THE CLITORIS: Whenever you are teasing a woman for the purpose of arousal, use all of her body as an erogenous zone and as much of her genitals as possible. Of course, the genitals are a perfect way to turn her on, so try stimulating the lips of her yoni. Tickle, rub, and wiggle one lip at a time or both sides simultaneously. Now and again, pretend you are going to give her what she wants (such as penetration), and even tell her so. Then do something else instead. After building excitement toward her clitoris, make her think you are just about to reach it, and then back off again. Ask her what she is craving, and tease her by telling her how you are going to satisfy her.

When the woman is sufficiently aroused, place the non-stimulating hand (palm down) flat against her pubic mound. Slide this hand toward her navel, stretching the hood off of the head and shaft of the clitoris. With the clitoris exposed, use the lubricated index and middle finger of your stimulating hand and begin direct stimulation of her clitoris. Once again, experiment to discover what she enjoys most. Be sure to ask her as well.

There are several variations for stroking the clitoris. Long or short strokes can be used. Up-and-down or side-to-side motions are possible. Making circles around the clitoris is another variation. Also try letting the movement come from the *wrist,* rather than the *finger* itself, or see if finger movements work best for you. All of these variations have their advantages and disadvantages.

STEP 5–BUILDING THE LEVELS OF ORGASM: Once you find the stroke your partner enjoys most, be sure to apply it as consistently as possible. When you feel an inevitable orgasm, slow down your touch, or change the direction until the orgasm slightly subsides. As the arousal level decreases, ask your partner to take a few deep breaths as she visualizes the orgasmic energy moving throughout her body. Then return to the preferred stimulation and again raise her level of arousal to the near point of orgasm. Once more bring her down and ask her to spread the energy throughout her body.

Whenever your partner gets close to an orgasm, pause and hold your fingers over the clitoral area. After several seconds, start the stroking again. Bring her up several times to where she almost cums. Then pause and hold the area (or have her channel the energy up through the spine) until the sensations calm down (de-tumesce). Begin the stimulation again to build tumescence and then de-tumesce once more.

You are obviously teasing your partner by building her up and then letting her calm down again. This develops energy, anticipation, and trust. However, there is a critical point where you have teased her enough, and it's time to take her through a well-deserved orgasm. At this point, she might be so aroused that she has more than one release–although this doesn't often happen the first time you stimulate the clitoris.

Be aware that in the early stages of sexual healing, some women cannot be repeatedly brought back and forth to the brink of orgasm. Instead, her body may be patterned to approach orgasm only once. In such instances, if her body doesn't climax, it refuses further stimulation often resulting in the loss of arousal. However, be patient and keep practicing.

STEP 6–THE ORGASMIC RELEASE: When your partner has reached the moment of inevitable orgasm, she should communicate that she is about to cum. Now more than ever, it's important to maintain the pace and pressure of the stimulation until it's obvious that she is ready to come down. You can assist in bringing her down by slowing and/or changing the stroke. The length of time you spend de-tumescing her can vary from a few seconds to several minutes. Be sure to tell her what you are doing, so she knows you are confident and in control.

After the woman's orgasms subside, and she comes down slightly, begin to stimulate the clitoris again, but be extra careful, as her clitoris might be ultra sensitive at this point.

After reaching and holding a plateau for a few moments, you can once again increase your partner's level of arousal. It's important to return to the strokes that she likes best and be sure you convey your own enjoyment with every stroke you give.

STEP 7–COMING DOWN: When it's time to completely de-tumesce your partner, be sure to communicate this to her. Gradually slow down the clitoral stimulation until you finally stop. Then place the stimulating hand over her yoni (palm down) and your other hand over her heart, while channeling energy between your two hands.

TECHNIQUE:
Pleasuring the G-spot

G-spot stimulation is known to be as pleasurable as clitoral stimulation but in quite a different way. It takes longer to arouse and is therefore often overlooked. When using the proper technique, **the G-spot can take a woman to levels of orgasm that clitoral orgasms can never reach.** But it's wise to awaken the clitoris and other parts of the yoni before approaching the G-spot. Once the woman is aroused enough, her G-spot begins to swell or engorge, which makes it easier to find. Some G-spots even engorge enough to become visible from the outside of the yoni.

It is commonly found that when stimulated, the G-spot adds pressure on the bladder and urethra, creating a sensation to urinate. However, if the woman has emptied her bladder, this urge is more likely the sensation of an upcoming ejaculation. Therefore, the woman should relax through the sensation to urinate, as the feeling will usually pass, or she will ejaculate. If the woman is too concerned, she can place some towels under her bottom in case she releases fluid. Nevertheless, if she relaxes, the sensation to urinate will give way to new levels of orgasm and pleasure.

Although the concept of sexual pain is often foreign to many women, some women experience physical and psychological pain during sexual intercourse. This discomfort stems from past negative experiences connected to their sexual histories. In such cases, the stimulation and resulting release of pressure from the G-spot can be a very emotional experience because the G-spot acts as a reservoir of sexual trauma and painful memories. In such cases, the woman's G-spot might even be painful to the touch. Ask her to take some deep breaths and relax as you gently massage the G-spot. She might experience emotional releases in the form of tears or anger, but remain calm, loving, and patient, as the emotions pass. She might feel the pain subside a little or even dissolve completely. While you are waiting patiently, mentally send lots of love into the G-spot area, and every so often, continue the stroking. Eventually, she will begin to feel pleasure. This transition from pain to pleasure could take one session or perhaps several.

STEP 1–CREATING A CONNECTION: Similar to the stimulation of the clitoris, the first step, after the woman empties her bladder and before stimulating the G-spot, is to connect with the woman's body by gently caressing her limbs and torso, always moving in the direction of the yoni.

In preparation, use plenty of pillows so that both of you are in comfortable positions. Next, place a towel underneath your partner, and place the lubricant (preferably water-based for the G-spot) nearby. Make sure the room is warm enough to eliminate the need for blankets. Prior to commencing contact with the G-spot, tease and stimulate the major and minor lips of the yoni, as well as awakening the clitoris.

STEP 2–CONTACTING THE G-SPOT: Many practitioners of sacred sexuality refer to this area as the "sacred spot." The size of the G-spot can range from that of a dime to a fifty-cent piece, and the location varies slightly from woman to woman. In most women, the G-spot is located about an inch inside the yoni on the upper wall. The area feels ridged and spongy and usually swells to a greater size during sexual arousal.

The first time you try to awaken the G-spot, remember it's common for a woman *not* to have an orgasm when this spot is initially stimulated. Nevertheless, keep your attention on loving and healing the sacred spot *and* on arousing the deep pleasure of your partner.

To contact the G-spot, let your secondary hand stimulate the woman's clitoris, while your primary hand slides beneath her tailbone (palm up). When it feels like she is yearning for it, insert the thumb of your primary hand into the opening of her yoni. Make circular motions with your thumb, awakening the inside of the yoni in all directions. You can now massage the inside of her yoni. Begin by rubbing two fingers along the floor of the vagina (directly opposite the G-spot). Move the fingers in and out along the vaginal floor, experimenting with massaging at different paces. This stimulates nerves embedded near the spinal cord and might help awaken and stimulate the woman's yoni.

Massage and arouse your partner using the techniques that "turn her on" the most. Continue massaging for a while before attempting to contact her sacred spot, and keep watching for signs of arousal. Once she has reached a high level of sexual excitement, ask if she is ready for you to work directly on her G-spot. When she is ready, insert either the ring and middle fingers or the index and middle fingers of your primary hand into the opening of the yoni (palm up), and press your fingertips carefully against her G-spot. Then begin gently massaging the entire G-spot from one side to the other and from front to back.

STEP 3–STIMULATING THE G-SPOT: Once you have made initial contact, curl your finger(s) against the G-spot with a moderate amount of pressure. Increase the pressure slowly and gradually until you reach a level of pressure the woman finds pleasing–which might change now and again. Watch her response to the pressure to help determine what she enjoys. Then begin moving your finger again and again in a beckoning ("come here") motion.

Continue the strokes in a steady manner, only one or two strokes per second, while encouraging her to breathe fully and include occasional "aaahhhh" sounds as she breathes. Pause periodically, relax, and then start again.

Although you can experiment with various strokes to stimulate the G-spot, the most common and effective technique is to slide your fingertips back and forth (from back to front) repetitively in the "come here" motion. Other variations of stimulating the G-spot include the following:

- Sliding your fingers in and out of the yoni and simultaneously rock your wrist side to side, which results in your fingers rubbing the G-spot thoroughly.
- Tapping the G-spot with your inserted finger.
- Stimulating the clitoris with one hand while you vibrate the G-spot with the fingers of your other hand.

STEP 4–BUILDING THE LEVELS OF ORGASM: Place your free hand (palm down) over the woman's pubic mound and just above her pubic bone. Press lightly into her body, as this pushes the G-spot down to meet your stimulating fingers. Once again (as with clitoral stimulation), be sure to observe her body's reactions and ask her to communicate when she approaches orgasm. Before she cums, slow down the pace of your stimulation and use your secondary hand to gently rock her lower abdomen back and forth. Ask her to breathe deeply and imagine spreading the orgasmic energy throughout her body. When the urge to orgasm passes, return to stimulation until another orgasm approaches, at which time you will again bring her down *before* she orgasms. As mentioned previously, this procedure can be done as many times as the woman desires. Yet, at the right moment, she can also be brought to orgasm.

STEP 5–THE ORGASMIC RELEASE: In the event the woman does not have a G-spot orgasm, reassure her that this is normal for most women. But emphasize that each pleasurable sensation she experienced *was* indeed a form of orgasm. On the other hand, if she *is* fortunate enough to have a G-spot orgasm, she should communicate when she is ready to release. As this moment arises, very slightly decrease the amount of pressure used until she releases and is well through the orgasm. Be aware that a G-spot orgasm can also release ejaculatory fluid. If this is the case, be sure to respond positively and encourage her to relax and allow it to happen.

STEP 6–COMING DOWN: Just as you would do after clitoral pleasuring, when it's time to de-tumesce your partner, communicate this to her. Gradually decrease stimulation to the G-spot until the de-tumescing feels complete. Now place the stimulating hand over her yoni (palm down) and your other hand over her heart while channeling energy between your two hands.

TECHNIQUE:
Combined Pleasuring of the Clitoris and G-spot

It must not be assumed that all women can easily reach orgasm with the combined pleasuring of the clitoris and G-spot and certainly not without practice. Yet for those who are willing to explore the possibility, combining clitoral and G-spot pleasuring to reach orgasm is summarized as follows: Stimulate the woman's clitoris in a manner that she enjoys most, until she is thoroughly aroused and approaches orgasm at least two or three times. Then insert two fingers into her yoni and begin massaging her G-spot, while continuing to stimulate her clitoris, until she nears orgasm a few more times. Finally, she is brought all the way through orgasm with the combined stimulation of her clitoris and G-spot. These can be done as simultaneous orgasms or alternating from one to the other.

STEP 1–CREATING A CONNECTION: Once again, as with the clitoral and G-spot exercises, it's important to create a loving, sensual connection before you commence pleasuring. Enhance this connection by using teasing and caressing touches throughout the woman's body in the direction of her yoni. While making connection, be sure to breathe deeply together, and give her verbal reminders to relax and let go.

STEP 2–CONTACTING THE CLITORIS AND G-SPOT: Apply oil-based lubricant to the clitoris and either oil or water-based lubricant to the major and minor lips of the yoni. Thoroughly massage the lips of the yoni in small circular motions, as well as gently pinching and fluttering the lips. Tease the index and middle fingers of your primary hand across the clitoris until the woman's pelvis begins to move.

STEP 3–STIMULATING THE CLITORIS AND G-SPOT: When enough arousal is achieved, slide those same two fingers into the opening of her yoni, and begin caressing her G-spot in a "come here" motion. When her body responds in a heightened state of arousal to the G-spot stimulation, let the thumb of your primary hand make contact once again with her clitoris. Allow your thumb to begin making strokes across the clitoris as your fingers caress the G-spot. Visualize an energetic connection between your stimulating fingers and thumb, which activates a connection between her clitoris and G-spot.

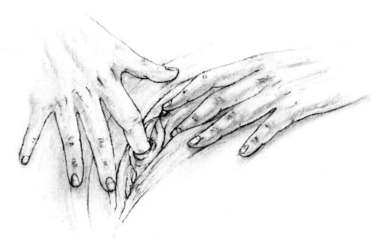

Pleasuring the clitoris and G-spot

You can also add stimulation to the clitoris with your passive hand, enhancing her arousal. Use the clitoris to bring her to a high state of pleasure again. Then hold those fingers still, and go back to the G-spot, stroking again for several minutes. Then return again to the clitoris.

Continue alternating between the clitoris and the G-spot several times. This alternating allows her body and mind to make an equal association between these two areas. The entire process of connecting the clitoris and G-spot should last about twenty minutes.

If you encounter resistance to stimulation from either the clitoris or G-spot, remain loving and patient–any other response suggests ulterior agendas. Work through resistance issues together. For some women, even with consistent practice, reaching a high level of orgasmic response can take months. Remember to pause regularly to allow the energy to spread throughout the woman's body. During the pauses, ask her to relax deeply and to occasionally shake her hips and limbs to release any pent-up energy. These pauses are very important, as continual stimulation can become too intense and even irritating. Furthermore, the pauses allow her to integrate the waves of pleasure.

STEP 4–BUILDING THE LEVELS OF ORGASM: After discovering the speed and pressure of the stroke that's most enjoyable to the woman, maintain that stroke until she approaches an orgasm. She should communicate when she is reaching an orgasm; at which time, you must slow the stimulation and ask her to take deep relaxing breaths while she mentally spreads the orgasmic energy through her body. After the arousal level has subsided, take her up and bring her down again several times until both of you agree that it's time for an orgasmic release.

An alternative technique for stimulating is to place your palm over your partner's yoni with your ring and middle fingers on the G-spot and the heel of that hand against the clitoris. Begin vibrating your hand, stimulating the clitoris and the G-spot at the same time. Maintain whatever pace of stimulation you choose until she is ready to reach orgasm. Then, de-tumesce her by slowing the pace and channeling energy through your palm into her yoni until the time feels right to build her up again for another orgasm. You can use this step at the start of the stimulation process (to assist arousal), during (to add to the buildup), or toward the end (to assist in spreading out the sensations, which are sometimes focused on the clitoris).

STEP 5–THE ORGASMIC RELEASE: When she finally releases a combined orgasm, have her use her breath, mind, and PC muscle to spread the orgasmic energy upward throughout her body as you continue a consistent pace of stimulation. When the orgasm has slightly subsided, slow the pace of your stimulation as well. When the time is right, take her up again for another orgasmic release. With some women the first release is the most intense, and the following orgasms are more subtle, wave-like sensations. Yet, for other women, the orgasms continue to become more intense after the first release. In either case, the goal is to eventually encourage the woman to become aware of her state of consciousness and the waves of energy expanding beyond her body.

If you find that your partner is having "squeeze contractions" (and is tightening, rather than relaxing, the muscles in her pelvis), begin stroking her G-spot with two fingers and mentally spreading out some of the ecstatic energy, while you encourage her to push the energy toward your palm. This technique might then help her to move into "push-out contractions." Afterwards, go back to the previous technique of stimulation, and lightly build arousal once again until she prepares for another orgasm. If she begins squeezing and pulling in, return to the G-spot technique just mentioned and spread out the energy again (encourage relaxing and pushing out) until she cums or the arousal subsides.

STEP 6–COMING DOWN: Once again, just as you would after clitoral or G-spot pleasuring, de-tumesce your partner. Gradually decrease stimulation to the clitoris and G-spot until the de-tumescing feels complete. Now place the G-spot stimulating hand over her yoni (palm down) and your clitoral stimulating hand over her heart, while channeling energy, love, and appreciation into these two centers of your partner.

IMPORTANT REMINDERS
FOR MANUALLY PLEASURING A WOMAN

- Manually pleasuring the clitoris or G-spot can be done separately or together.
- The stroke preference varies from one woman to another, as does the amount of preferred pressure. Start lightly and gradually increase until you find the best pressure.
- For manually pleasuring a woman, use the pad of the finger, rather than the tip.
- Anchoring the clitoris *against* your thumb or between your thumb and forefinger will keep the clitoris from slipping away from the touch of the other hand.
- Use a consistent, steady stroke to arouse your partner to the first peak. As long as the sensation keeps building, continue the same stroke.
- Let her know how great it feels to touch her and watch her being pleasured. Also, remember to compliment her, especially when you observe any signs of orgasms–small or large.
- There are two important, basic strokes for stimulating the clitoris: (1) short up-and-down strokes directly over the clitoris and (2) small circular motions around the clitoris. Either of these two strokes (alone or combined) are enough to excite your partner to orgasm. But take time to discover new strokes and incorporate them as well.

Manually Pleasuring a Man

Men are often accused of being obsessed with their lingams. Despite the image, many men are self-conscious about having their lingams thoroughly pleasured. They would much prefer a quickie "hand job" that allows them to remain free of intimacy and vulnerability. Nevertheless, encourage your partner to lie back, receive, and allow *you* to be in charge. The more you sense his rush to get to the goal line, the more you should back off and de-tumesce him. This, of course, is not meant to be cruel, but rather to assist him in learning self-discipline and understanding sacred sexuality, which in turn, assists in his evolution.

TECHNIQUE:

Pleasuring the Lingam

Although it only takes a short stroke to run the entire length of a clitoris, the lingam needs longer strokes to achieve full stimulation. There are numerous techniques for massaging a lingam, but the person doing the pleasuring should discover not only what her partner likes but also what feels comfortable for her *own* hands. One of the most common techniques is to grip the base of the lingam with one hand and massage the shaft of the lingam with the other hand, using as much surface area of the hand as possible. The massaging hand should pay special attention to the underside of the lingam, where the greatest amount of sensation is felt.

The entire lingam contains many nerve endings, so be sure to massage its entire length. To stimulate a man to intense peaks of arousal, begin your strokes with a fairly firm grip near the base but lighten this grip as you get close to the head of the lingam. Focus on the sensations in your hands. Feel the texture of his lingam against your fingertips and palms, and notice how it makes you feel inside.

As the person doing the pleasuring, take control of the lovemaking and encourage your partner to relax and not think about anything. However, communication is important, so be sure to ask him to let you know when he is about to cum. This is something you eventually need to practice sensing on your own.

With experience and the development of intuition, you will discover how far you can take your partner without bringing him to ejaculation. The farther he has gone into the ejaculation phase, the more difficult it will be to pause and shift into practicing an in-jaculation, or other levels of orgasm. Later, of course, you might agree that it's time to let him ejaculate.

To increase the effects of an in-jaculation, a man must develop the ability to become as stimulated as possible without ejaculating, or remain on the safe side of the "point of no return." As he reaches this limit and gives you the signal, slow down, change what you're doing, and slightly decrease his level of arousal. It should only take thirty seconds for the sensation of ejaculation to pass. The more times he refrains from cumming and channels his energy, the more the energy will build for the moment he finally decides to release.

STEP 1–CREATING A CONNECTION: Before pleasuring a male, first connect with him by rubbing his shoulders, sitting on his lap, and perhaps giving him long hugs and kisses. Eventually, take a moment to gaze into his eyes and synchronize your breathing with his. Then invite him to sit or lie back and relax.

Begin stroking and teasing his body with your fingers, hair, and breasts. Use these various body parts to make long stroking movements toward his lingam. If he seems to resist relaxing, give him an unexpected, playful nibble or an occasional bite to help him lighten-up.

STEP 2–CONTACTING THE LINGAM: When contacting the erect penis, use plenty of the appropriate lubricant. To make initial contact with the lingam, begin by stroking your fingertips from his perineum to his scrotum. Do this several times before you eventually allow your hand to continue the stroke onto the lingam from the base to the tip.

STEP 3–STIMULATING THE LINGAM: There are numerous techniques for stimulating the male lingam. The best hand stroke is the one that feels best between you and your partner. However, there are a few simple strokes that are the most popular. They are as follows:

- One Hand Stroke–Hold the base of the lingam (above the scrotum) with one hand, while the other hand makes long repetitive strokes up and down the full length of the lingam. Since the underside of the lingam is the most sensitive (especially just below the head), be mindful to stimulate this area.

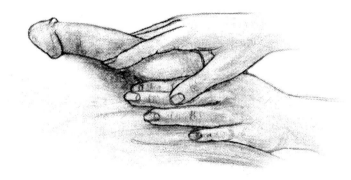

One hand stroke

- Two Hand Stroke–Slide one hand from the base to the tip of the lingam, and just as it completes the stroke, have the other hand begin to stroke from the base to the tip. Stroke from the base of the lingam to the head and back down again. Continue these strokes, alternating from one hand to the other, while observing the man's response–particularly in the movement of his pelvis and thighs.

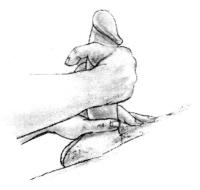

Two hand stroke

- Churning Butter–Clasp both hands together with palms facing each other and fingers interlaced. Slightly separate your palms and thumbs enough to create enough space for the lingam to slide between them. Then, slide your hands up and down along the lingam. Don't slide too fast or you'll quickly tire your arms. Besides, a faster stroke is not necessarily better. Also, alternate a few short strokes to one long stroke.

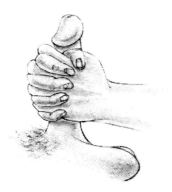

Churning butter

STEP 4–BUILDING THE LEVELS OF ORGASM: After you have pleasured your partner's lingam with various hand (and/or mouth) techniques and have discovered which one brings him the greatest pleasure, continue using that technique. Gradually raise his level of arousal until he approaches orgasm. Before he reaches his point of no return, begin to slow your stroke, move your hand beneath the scrotum to the perineum, and begin to deeply massage the area until his arousal subsides. Encourage him to let you know when his point of no return draws near.

Once the man's arousal has slightly subsided, return to his favorite lingam stroke. Once again build his level of arousal, and then bring him down again. This process can be repeated several times to raise his overall level of ecstatic energy.

STEP 5–THE ORGASMIC RELEASE: Once you both decide that it's time for the man to experience an orgasmic release, you can bring him all the way through his orgasm. During his release, encourage him to inhale deeply as he channels the energy upward through his body to the top of his head. Then, he should exhale slowly and allow the energy to pour down the front of his body until it reaches his navel.

STEP 6–COMING DOWN: When it's time to completely de-tumesce your partner, be sure to communicate this to him. Gradually slow down the stimulation until you finally stop. Then place the stimulating hand over his lingam (palm down) and your other hand over his heart and channel energy between your two hands.

TECHNIQUE:

Pleasuring the Prostate

Pleasuring the prostate can be done either externally (through the perineum) or internally (through the anus). Stimulating the prostate is the male equivalent of stimulating the G-spot. It can create explosive, new levels of orgasm for the man and helps to keep the prostate healthy. **A prostate orgasm creates a more *internal*, energetic orgasm, as opposed to the more *external* explosion of a physical, lingam orgasm.**

Be sure to communicate with your partner and watch his reactions. Direct contact with the male's sacred spot (prostate gland) is done by inserting a finger into the rectum and hooking it forward towards the abdomen–just like the primary technique for massaging a woman's G-spot. Of course both partners need to be mindful of certain necessary precautions. First, they must both be comfortable doing such a vulnerable technique. Second, the rectum should be empty and clean. Third, nothing that makes contact with the rectum should have contact with any other orifice–especially the vagina–without a thorough washing. Some lovers choose to use finger condoms or surgical gloves for anal contact, as they are more sanitary and can be removed.

STEP 1–CREATING A CONNECTION: Before pleasuring a male, first connect with him by rubbing his shoulders, sitting on his lap, and giving him long hugs and kisses. Take a moment to gaze into his eyes and synchronize your breathing with his. Then invite him to lie back and relax. Now, to ease his resistance and physical tensions, massage his thighs, low back, and buttocks muscles.

STEP 2–CONTACTING THE PROSTATE: To contact the prostate from the outside, first lubricate the perineum thoroughly with an oil-based or silicone lubricant, and then begin gently massaging the region. Gradually decrease the surface area being rubbed to a point directly between the scrotum and anus. To make deeper contact, press with either your fingers or the knuckles of your fist, and begin massaging deeply into this area. It might create sensations of mild discomfort but only because this region is unaccustomed to manual stimulation. When pressing deeply, stimulate with either small circular motions, back and forth movements, and/or hand vibration. Continue stimulating the prostate (through the perineum) for about five to ten minutes. If you and your partner decide to stimulate the prostate through the *anus*, be sure to use non-latex gloves.

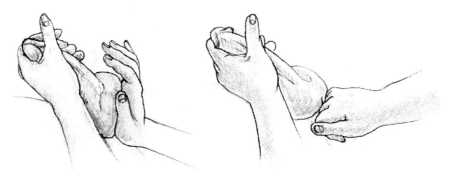

Pleasuring the prostate

STEP 3–STIMULATING THE PROSTATE: As with the *external* prostate massage, begin by rubbing the perineum area and gradually move to the anus. Using plenty of lubricant, gently slide your index or middle finger (a little at a time) into the anus and curl the finger towards his navel. If you sense any resistance or tightening, pause and back off very slightly until you feel the anal muscles relax before you proceed further. When your finger is inserted approximately two inches, the pad of your finger (turned towards the naval) should be able to feel the aroused prostate gland. Begin massaging the prostate with your finger in a "come here" motion.

Stimulating the prostate gland can cause slight discomfort, especially when the man has not experienced this before. If the discomfort is excessive, he should have an exam to check the health of his prostate. But even if the prostate stimulation feels good to the man, the massage should not exceed five to ten minutes; otherwise, it could begin to feel irritating.

If the prostate massage is pleasurable, try a few different prostate massage techniques. As with G-spot massage, you can experiment with various strokes to stimulate the prostate. The most common and effective technique is to slide your fingertip back and forth (from back to front) repetitively in the "come here" motion. Other variations include:

- Sliding your finger forward and backward as you simultaneously rock your wrist side to side, which results in your fingers rubbing the prostate thoroughly.
- Tapping the prostate with your inserted finger.
- Stimulating the lingam with one hand while you vibrate the prostate with the finger of your other hand.

STEP 4–BUILDING THE LEVELS OF ORGASM: The prostate is much like a woman's G-spot. Therefore, stimulation of the prostate is different from that of the lingam, as is the difference between stimulation of the G-spot and clitoris. Find a massage technique that brings the most pleasure and use it to arouse your partner to near orgasm. As with all methods of building an orgasm, once he gets close to cumming, slow your touch, and bring him down. After a few moments, increase the stimulation again. When he is close to orgasm, repeat the de-tumescing process by slowing down or holding still.

STEP 5–THE ORGASMIC RELEASE: When it's time for your partner to experience an orgasmic release of the prostate, encourage him to inhale deeply through his mouth and then, as he exhales, he should push the energy downward toward his pelvis. He needs to push downward only enough to keep his pelvic and genital muscles from contracting. This downward push will create a sensation of losing control (perhaps of his bladder) but continue the stimulation until your partner has an orgasm.

STEP 6–COMING DOWN: Just as you would do after lingam pleasuring, when it's time to de-tumesce your partner, communicate this to him. Gradually decrease stimulation to the prostate until the de-tumescing feels complete. After cleaning your hands, place the stimulating hand over his groin (palm down) and your other hand over his heart, while channeling energy between your two hands.

TECHNIQUE:
Combined Pleasuring of the Lingam and Prostate

A man may have experienced sexual "heights" in his life, which may have been accomplished through shallow and rushed forms of sex. However, **when he experiences the "depths" of sex, which is brought about in part by practicing lengthier forms of lovemaking, such as combined lingam and prostate pleasuring, he will never be the same.**

The process of reaching orgasm by combining lingam and prostate pleasuring can be summarized as follows: Stimulate his lingam until he is clearly aroused. Then add stimulation to the perineum with a light, then firm, touch until he is brought near to orgasm at least two or three times. Next, insert a finger into his anus and begin directly massaging his prostate, while still manually stimulating his lingam, until he is brought close to orgasm a few more times. Finally, he is brought all the way through orgasm with the combined stimulation of his lingam and prostate.

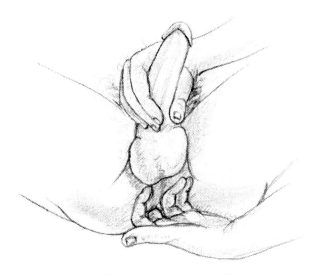

Pleasuring the lingam and prostate

STEP 1–CREATING A CONNECTION: After you have had enough experience individually pleasuring your partner's lingam and prostate, you can combine the pleasuring of both. To do so involves the use of most of the individual exercises for pleasuring the lingam or prostate. However, before you begin any pleasuring, it is important to create a connection by breathing together, communicating, and sharing loving, physical contact.

STEP 2–CONTACTING THE LINGAM AND PROSTATE: The first step is to stimulate the lingam. This intimate, sensuous contact allows the man to begin the process of releasing, relaxing, and trusting. After he relaxes into the arousal, start massaging his perineum gently and then more deeply towards the prostate. Next, penetrate the anus with one finger from your secondary hand. Then, with the other (primary) hand, begin stimulating his lingam (using plenty of lubricant).

STEP 3–STIMULATING THE LINGAM AND PROSTATE: While holding the secondary hand still (with the pad of your finger on the prostate), vigorously stimulate the lingam with your primary hand. Once your partner reaches a heightened state of arousal (which he should communicate), gently begin caressing his prostate gland, while continuing the stimulation of his lingam. This will create a simultaneous arousal in both the lingam and prostate.

STEP 4–BUILDING THE LEVELS OF ORGASM: It's important to find the pace and pressure of stimulation that gives your partner the most pleasure. Experiment with various styles of touch on the prostate. Try rubbing in a "come here" motion, tapping with the pad of your finger, rubbing in a circular motion, or vibrating the prostate with the pad of your finger. Once you find the technique your partner enjoys most, continue with combined pleasuring of the prostate and lingam, bringing your partner nearer to a state of ecstatic orgasm.

As he approaches the point of no return, slow the pace of stimulation of your *primary* hand, and then hold steady. Apply deep pressure on the prostate with your *secondary* hand and encourage your partner to inhale slowly and deeply, decreasing his level of arousal. After a few moments of deeper but slower stimulation, you can again increase your partner's level of arousal and continue this cycle until you both agree it's time for an orgasm.

STEP 5–THE ORGASMIC RELEASE: When it's time for your partner to have a combined orgasmic release, it should be obvious that the ecstatic energy has filled his entire pelvic region, as well as his abdomen and thighs. Then, it's time to bring him through the orgasm. Ask him to inhale slowly and deeply through his mouth and to relax all his muscles, particularly those in his pelvis. Stimulate your partner's lingam and prostate until he cums. Afterward, he will feel waves of ecstatic pleasure streaming through his body. He may or may not ejaculate. Either way, reduce the pace of stimulation to the lingam and prostate while these orgasmic waves continue.

STEP 6–COMING DOWN: Once again, just as you would do after lingam or prostate pleasuring, it's now time to de-tumesce your partner. Gradually decrease stimulation to the lingam and prostate until the de-tumescing feels complete. After cleaning your hands, place one hand over your partner's groin (palm down) and your other hand over his heart, while channeling energy, love, and appreciation into these two centers of your partner.

IMPORTANT REMINDERS
FOR MANUALLY PLEASURING A MAN

- Manually pleasuring the lingam or prostate can be done separately or together.
- The stroke preference varies from one man to another, as does the amount of preferred pressure. Most men enjoy steady, firm strokes.
- Use a consistent, steady stroke to arouse your partner to the first peak. As long as the sensation keeps building, continue the same stroke.
- Let him know how great it feels to touch him and watch him being pleasured. Remember to compliment him, especially when you observe any signs of orgasm–small or large.
- For the best results when pleasuring a partner, remember to tease him with actions and words. Keeping your strokes steady and repetitive will help you stay connected to your lover–which encourages him to surrender to you and allows you to take him higher.
- Keep in mind that signs of orgasm can take many forms–even slight surges. Accept and appreciate the smaller sensations and more will be added as the body is retrained.

Pleasuring the Anus
(The Shadow Spot)

Because of the phobias related to hygienic issues, germs, and inhibitions, the anus is one of the least explored erogenous zones. In fact, anal sex is illegal in some states and countries. Furthermore, when most women experience anal sex, it is often done to satisfy her partners' secret fetish or perhaps as an act of aggressive or experimental sex, more than for their own pleasure. So, it's no wonder that anal stimulation is a rarely explored **part of sexuality.**

It might be appropriate to begin using a new term for the anus, such as the "shadow spot." This is befitting since the "shadow" of a person's psyche is commonly thought to represent the darker, edgier aspects of our being; It represents the part of us we don't like others to see, as well as the parts they usually prefer not to see.

Nevertheless, the *shadow spot* is an erogenous zone and can be highly stimulating when explored. Although stimulation of the shadow spot need not progress to greater penetration, some people do prefer to explore anal contact as part of foreplay before proceeding to genital contact, as anal stimulation can arouse the body and remove inhibitions. Yet others prefer to start with the genitals, get them stimulated, proceed to the perineum for a while (teasing toward the anus), and finally move on to the shadow spot.

If you choose to do any form of anal stimulation, be sure your fingernails are well trimmed. Using plenty of lubricant, start by massaging the outer portion of the shadow spot for a while with an occasional tease of finger entry. Explore the center rim of the anal opening using a clock-face for a reference. Twelve o'clock is the part of the anus closest to the genitals. Massage each hour's spot for at least a quarter of a minute. Ask for feedback so that you can discover which part has proven to be most sensitive. Once discovered, you can occasionally return to this spot during any other lovemaking sessions with your partner. For example, sneak up on it once in a while when you are sharing oral pleasure.

Despite the many pleasures anal sex brings to some people, it is advisable not to probe the anus, rectum, and colon too often or with objects that are too long or wide. Such practices tend to confuse the natural peristalsis (direction of flow), as well as break down the tone of the inner tissue and the ring muscle.

TECHNIQUE:
Anal Pleasuring

Despite the many taboos against all forms of anal pleasuring, anal stimulation can result in more overall relaxation, which means less stress on the sexual organs and surrounding muscles. This reduction of tension translates to greater forms of release and less chance of premature ejaculation for the male. Anal pleasuring also allows direct stimulation of the prostate gland, which can create the same unique orgasmic pleasure as that of the female G-spot.

STEP 1: Prepare ahead by emptying the colon and bladder before an anal healing massage. Always sanitize the hands before and after anal contact.

STEP 2: Begin by lubricating your hands and the area around the perineum and anus. Then make initial contact by sensually teasing the outer portion of the perineum and anus.

STEP 3: When the time feels right for both of you, slowly and gently penetrate the anus with one finger. The depth of a finger's probe can vary based on your partner's level of excitement, stimulation, and feedback. The average depth of exploration is to the first knuckle (or about an inch). The techniques can vary from insertion/withdrawal, wiggling, and rubbing the anal rim with the pad of the finger.

STEP 4: As you continue the anal massage, remind your partner to breathe deeply and slowly to relax any tensions that might arise. As he or she does so, vibrate the inserted finger or rub any tender area. As you penetrate a little deeper, you will find some areas of discomfort, such as the prostate, tailbone, or sacrum. In such cases, always focus on sending healing energy to the painful area as you massage gently.

STEP 5: If the choice is made to stimulate the prostate, make sure your finger is well lubricated, and insert your finger about two inches (pad up) as your partner lies on his back. Then, with the same technique that is used to massage the female's G-spot, massage upward towards his navel with a "come here" motion.

STEP 6: When it's time to conclude, ask your partner's permission to withdraw your finger. Then sanitize your hands, not from shame associated with the anus, but to remove any germs.

STEP 7: Allow your partner time to relax and integrate the experience. It's best not to have intercourse immediately after anal massage.

CHAPTER 14

Oral Sex

Making Love Using Your Mouth

Although oral sex is considered taboo by some, the ancients taught that oral sex is a delightful addition to any sexual experience. **When practiced correctly, oral sex can be *at least* as pleasurable as intercourse itself.** In the arts of sacred sex, there are several recommended techniques for orally pleasuring a man or a woman.

Like mouth kissing, oral sex has numerous variations. It can be experienced as a part of foreplay or complete in itself. Oral pleasuring is a wonderful gift from one person to another or as a simultaneous exchange.

Despite the taboos, there are rewarding aspects to oral pleasuring and ejaculation ingestion. For example, the fluids ejaculated by a male (which average one teaspoon) are high in protein, life-promoting energy, antibiotic properties, and nutrients, including vitamin C, iron, and calcium. The nutrients in a teaspoon of semen are said to equal two steaks, ten eggs, and several oranges combined–not to mention vital energy. Semen, therefore, can be healthy to ingest. Since these nutrients come from the man's body, however, each ejaculation depletes his endocrine glands unless proper techniques are utilized to magnify and retain the otherwise lost vital essence and nutrients.

Performing cunnilingus or fellatio is said to exercise and tone the facial muscles and strengthen the gum tissue.

Before engaging in oral sex, it is advisable that the genitals be as clean as possible and "protection" be considered. Also, the partner pleasuring should have a clean mouth. Cleanliness cuts down on the number of potential germs being transferred. You might use a dental dam (available in flavors) or kitchen cellophane. Of course, these germs become less of a concern if you and your partner have a long-term, monogamous relationship.

There are a few important reminders for orally pleasuring a woman or man. They are as follows:

- Orally pleasuring the yoni or lingam can be combined with manually pleasuring other parts of the sexual anatomy.
- The preferred oral technique varies from person to person. Be sure to ask what your partner likes and learn by observation.
- When you notice your partner reaching the point of orgasm, unless you want him or her to cum, be sure to alter your stimulation to something less arousing until the urge subsides.
- Use moans and gentle body movements to let your partner know how great you feel when you are pleasuring him or her.

Cunnilingus: Orally Pleasuring a Woman

The oral pleasuring of a man to a woman is commonly referred to as *cunnilingus*, meaning "to pleasure the cunni (yoni) with the lingual, tongue." When pleasuring a woman, never proceed directly to the clitoris. Instead, tease her and build up her arousal by first pleasuring *other* parts of her body and genitals. When you finally connect with the clitoris, don't devour it! Play with it gently. Lightly touch and lick around and across it. Besides licking, there can also be some sucking. But it's important to refrain from sucking the clitoris too hard, or you might hurt it and make your lover feel more numbness than arousal. You might also include playing with the clitoral legs.

If you are performing cunnilingus for the first time on a partner (or if you feel insecure about it), begin by licking the outer lips and progressing to the inner lips. Let your hands assist to spread the yoni's lips apart). The licking motion, at first, looks similar to licking an ice-cream cone. Then it progresses to such various tongue motions as side-to-side, faster flicking, and even a stiffening of the tongue for insertion into the yoni.

You need not worry about being an anatomy expert, just experiment with different techniques and use them on various parts of your partner's yoni. As you practice orally pleasuring your lover and communicating with her, you will discover what techniques work best.

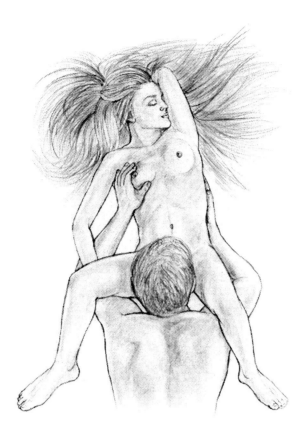

Orally pleasuring a woman

There are numerous variations for pleasuring a woman, including the following:

- The woman stands, tilting her yoni forward so you can reach her with your tongue.
- Use vertical and horizontal strokes across her clitoris.
- Use variations of pleasuring with the tip and flat of your tongue.
- For triple stimulation, stimulate her clitoris with your tongue, while also stimulating her G-spot with one hand and her nipples with the other.
- Alternate taking warm tea and cold ice into your mouth while pleasuring her.
- Rest your upper lip on her *mons* and slowly swirl your tongue clockwise from clitoris to lips.

THE THREE SECRETIONS
FROM THE PEAKS OF AROUSAL

When orally pleasuring a woman, think of it as exchanging love, energy, and essences. The ancients taught that saliva mixed with yoni juice creates nectar that nourishes both partners. They encouraged the male to drink deeply of the woman's love juices because they are healing, nurturing, and rejuvenating. Absorption of the yoni juices and the accompanying energetic essences takes place through the mouth and/or penis. Taoist sexual masters teach that the two primary ways for the male to maintain youthful vitality are to retain semen and/or to absorb the woman's essence (juice) orally and via the lingam. The latter is practiced by the male placing his lingam inside his partner while imagining he is soaking up, or absorbing, her love juices through his lingam–like sipping through a straw.

When absorbing (or considering the importance of absorbing) the bodily secretions of your partner, remember that there is a difference between body *excretions* and sexual *secretions*. Bodily *excretions* are eliminated waste products, while sexual *secretions*, on the other hand, are life-giving fluids rich in nutrients and energy. Taoist sexologists teach that there are "Three Peaks" that offer *three secretions* (or yin essences). These are as follows:

1. The first is called the *High Peak* (or Red Lotus Peak), which offers frothy saliva that enters a woman's mouth from under her tongue.
2. The second is called the *Middle Peak* (or Twin Peaks), which offers a whitish, sweet secretion that comes from her breasts.
3. The third is called the *Lower Peak* (or Dark Gate Peak), which offers a thick secretion that comes from her yoni.

To absorb the woman's essence orally, practice pleasuring her and notice the saliva that fills your mouth. Mix this saliva with the yoni essence. Then, blend the two into a special elixir and drink deeply. A word of caution–before engaging in any direct sexual contact between the mouth and sexual organs, there are emotional, hygienic, and health factors that should be considered. Any signs or symptoms suggesting the lack of optimum health should be considered as safety warnings.

TECHNIQUE:

Orally Pleasuring a Woman

When pleasuring a man, it's the *technique* that first begins to soften his defenses. When pleasuring a woman, it's all about the *feeling*. If she is not physically and emotionally comfortable, it greatly diminishes the effects of the sensations. Therefore, make it a priority to open your heart and pleasure her from a place of love and caring.

STEP 1–CREATING A CONNECTION: Before orally pleasuring a woman, create a comfortable environment and establish a personal connection. Encourage her to lie back and breathe slowly and deeply as you gently caress her body. Tell her how beautiful she looks and how much you care for her. This loving attention will gradually seduce her legs open, at which time you can slide between her thighs. You may have to occasionally remind her to relax and let go.

STEP 2–CONTACTING THE YONI: Before your tongue makes contact *and* throughout the pleasuring session, let your fingers assist the arousal process. When it's time to make oral contact, you can do so with or without flavored oil.

STEP 3–ORALLY STIMULATING THE YONI: When it's clear that the woman is aroused and craving greater contact, let your tongue make teasing passes. Slide your tongue along the ridge of the outer lips and then the inner lips of the yoni. Move your tongue in either the direction of the clitoris or towards the opening of the yoni, as this increases the woman's anticipation. Add to her pleasure by licking her perineum.

Eventually let your tongue shift from longer, slower strokes to occasional quick flits, especially around the clitoris. Then surprise your lover by plunging your stiffened tongue into her yoni, curl the tip upward, and withdraw it, thus making contact with the G-spot. Eventually, replace the tongue thrusts with placing your thumb or finger against the G-spot as you begin focusing most of your oral pleasuring on her clitoris.

Alternate your tongue movements, as well as the body-part you are pleasuring. Notice what she enjoys the most, and gradually spend more time on that technique.

Remember to pause now and then to allow the sexual energy to spread throughout the woman's body. During the pauses, ask her to take a deep breath followed by an exhale as she slightly shakes her hips and limbs to release any pent-up energy. This will spread out her ecstatic energy, release tensions, and allow her to integrate the waves of pleasure.

STEP 4–BUILDING THE LEVELS OF ORGASM: Your partner might prefer being taken through an orgasm, or she may want to build to deeper levels of orgasm. If she is open to the latter, begin using the tempo and pressure of licking that proved most enjoyable to her. As she approaches orgasm, (which she should communicate), slow down your stimulation and move to pleasuring other, less stimulating areas, until her arousal slightly subsides. At this time, she should stroke her body with her fingertips, and mentally spread the orgasmic energy throughout her body. After the arousal level has subsided, take her up and bring her down again several times, until the time feels right for her to release an orgasm.

STEP 5–THE ORGASMIC RELEASE: When your oral pleasuring brings your lover to an orgasm, she should use her breath, mind, and PC muscle to spread the orgasmic energy upward throughout her body, as you slow your pace of stimulation. Be especially careful licking the clitoris during orgasm, as it tends to become hypersensitive. When the orgasm has slightly subsided, take her up again for another orgasmic release. If her clitoris remains too sensitive, move to other parts of the yoni. You may need to let your fingers assist you with pleasuring the G-spot, as this might bring your lover *another* type of orgasm. If so, touch and lick her G-spot until she releases again. Then, you can move back to clitoral pleasuring.

STEP 6–COMING DOWN: Once your partner has had one or several orgasms, it's time to de-tumesce her. Encourage your lover to become aware of waves of energy streaming though her body. Place one hand over her yoni (palm down) and your other hand over her heart, while channeling energy, love, and appreciation into these two centers of your partner.

IMPORTANT REMINDERS
FOR ORALLY PLEASURING A WOMAN

- Orally pleasuring the clitoris and yoni can be combined with manually pleasuring the G-spot.
- The preferred oral technique varies from one woman to another. So be sure to ask what your partner likes and learn by observation.
- When you notice your partner reaching the point of orgasm, unless

you want her to cum, be sure to alter your stimulation to something less arousing until her urge subsides.

• Use moans and gentle body movements to let her know how great you feel when you are pleasuring her.

Fellatio–Orally Pleasuring a Man

The oral pleasuring of a woman to a man is commonly referred to as *fellatio*, which comes from the word *phallic*, a term for a penis shaped object. A more common, but ignorant, term for this form of pleasuring a man is "blow job." Besides the obvious lack of tact, there is NO "blowing" involved in fellatio. This slang comes from an old English phrase that refers to a sexual act/favor (a "job") performed on a man by a prostitute, or "blo," as they were sometimes called. Hence the term "blo-job." Thus, it's understandable why this term might be considered disrespectful to a woman, as it equates her actions with that of a prostitute.

If you are new at (or insecure about) performing fellatio, begin by assessing your attitude toward performing this act. **The lingam is an extension of your lover that is capable of sending waves of pleasure and delightful sensations throughout his body.** If you treat this part of his body, as well as the act of fellatio with respect and reverence, oral pleasuring can take you both to new heights of vulnerability and arousal. If, on the other hand, you lack feelings of love, respect, and reverence when practicing fellatio, you should reconsider the act and perhaps the relationship as well.

Oral sex is a natural part of lovemaking. It can be an important addition to foreplay or stand alone as an act of lovemaking. Oral sex can also add another dimension of playfulness to sexual encounters. The very idea of a woman being coerced into performing fellatio is tragic. Yet, when a woman chooses to play the submissive role of pleasuring her partner, it can be one of the most amazing aspects of any sexual experience. Her submissiveness is a choice, not the result of being controlled, and she takes pleasure in the role she performs. When a woman properly performs oral sex, it may appear that she is submissive and exclusively in the role of giving. But, in reality, she too gains from the experience, as her partner reaches deep levels of vulnerability and she receives his life-enriched juice. Furthermore, *she* is the one who is in control. *She* will decide how much pleasure he feels and if and when he will be brought to orgasm.

The best position for performing fellatio is the most comfortable position for both partners. Yet, besides physical comfort, choose a position that creates a visual turn-on for the man. Then, while performing fellatio, be sure to look up at your lover. It creates an erotic visual scene for him to behold. The ideal is to magnify the man's excitement through mental (visual), as well as physical, stimulation. The visual stimulation evokes a mental orgasm to coincide with the physical and energetic orgasms. The woman can also add to the man's excitement by making faint moans of desire and sounds that beg for his lingam. While performing fellatio, produce as much saliva as possible–the more saliva the better. It creates a sensual lubricant for him, while producing protection against some bacteria and viruses. Another great turn-on for the man during fellatio is for him to place his hands on the head of his partner, hence the term, "giving head." This gives him a feeling of control, which, of course, is something he enjoys. If the pleasure gets too intense and the man becomes too forceful with his hand placement, tactfully remind him to be more gentle.

Before you begin oral pleasuring, experiment with placing a cool mint in your mouth. It adds a burst of stimulation to the lingam. When you begin pleasuring your partner's lingam, do so with licking motions (as on an ice-cream cone). Try variations of fast and slow licks. Then, when the time feels right, occasionally slide his lingam into and out of your mouth, making sure to avoid contact with your teeth. Use your lips to cover your teeth. Insert the lingam into your mouth a few times before returning to licking. Continue this cycle of licking and inserting as many times as you like. When you are ready, move on to intercourse or continue to pleasure your lover with any of the fellatio techniques described in this book or developed on your own. Be aware that it's mostly the insertion (rather than licking) that will bring your partner to orgasm. Pleasuring to the point of orgasm should occur only when you are both ready and it's mutually agreeable.

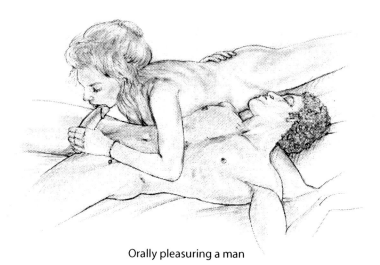

Orally pleasuring a man

There are several ways a woman can pleasure a man. Many of the ancient cultures have colorful names and descriptions for each technique. Some of the most common variations include the following:

1. Biting–The lingam is held and gentle bitten along the side.

2. Kissing–The lingam is licked and kissed as if it were the lips of her beloved.

3. Pressing–The lingam is brought into the mouth and withdrawn, back and forth.

4. Rotating–The lingam is brought into the mouth and licked and sucked as the mouth is rotated.

5. Rubbing–The lingam is rubbed all over with the tongue and lips.

6. Stroking–The lingam is held only part way into the mouth as the hand moves back and forth along the shaft.

7. Sucking–The lingam is brought halfway into the mouth and then sucked firmly as it is withdrawn.

8. Swallowing–The lingam is drawn in as far as is comfortable. Then the lips are extended forward to embrace more of the lingam, and the lingam is slowly drawn outward.

There are other variations of techniques for orally pleasuring a man including:

1. One hand on his lingam slides *towards* your mouth as your mouth slides down on the lingam.

2. One hand on his lingam slides *away* from your mouth as your mouth slides down on the lingam.

3. Take only the head of the lingam into your mouth and shake your head from side to side.

4. Cradle and massage your partner's testicles as you pleasure his lingam.

5. Occasionally suck on your partner's scrotum while you stroke him with your hand.

6. Have your partner stand up while you pleasure him. Also, place your hands on the back of his buttocks to pull him towards you.

7. Suck on the tip of your partner's lingam while you stroke the shaft of his lingam with your hand.

8. For triple stimulation, place the tip of your partner's lingam in your mouth while you stroke his shaft with one hand and massage his testicles with your other hand.

9. Guide your partner in and out of your mouth as you nod your head in "yes" fashion.

10. Alternately drink hot tea and suck on ice cubes in between orally pleasuring your partner.

11. A little clove oil can be rubbed under the ridge of the head of your partner's lingam. It slightly desensitizes the area that could otherwise cause a pre-mature ejaculation.

TECHNIQUE:
Orally Pleasuring a Man

When orally pleasuring a man, there are choices to be made of what you can do with the ejaculated fluids. You can either help him ejaculate into a tissue or towel or let him ejaculate onto any portion of your body. You can allow him to cum in your mouth and then tactfully spit it out, or you can choose to swallow the fluids of his ejaculation. Considering the possibility of STD's, the first two choices are the safest. The third choice is questionably safe, since it is believed that if semen is exposed to oxygen, it cannot transmit most viruses.

STEP 1–CREATING A CONNECTION: Before orally pleasuring a man, it's important to make him feel as though you crave him. As he stands, sits or lies back, ask him to close his eyes and take some deep breaths. Then rub and claw his skin in the direction of his genitals.

STEP 2–CONTACTING THE LINGAM: Slide your hand to your

partner's groin. If he has pants on, you can rub his stiffening penis more firmly. Otherwise, stroke it tenderly (at first) from end to end. Pause occasionally and grab the base of the shaft and give it a squeeze.

STEP 3–ORALLY STIMULATING THE LINGAM: By now, you should have your partner undressed. You may or may not choose to apply flavored oil to his lingam. When it's clear that he is fully aroused and erect, kneel or sit at his feet and begin oral contact by licking his perineum and scrotum. Gradually slide your tongue along the lingam, from base to tip. Do this several times, building his anticipation. Then surprise him by sliding your mouth onto his lingam and withdrawing it. Repeat this only a few times. He is sure to respond and want more, but make him wait. Eventually you can focus more time on the actual oral pleasuring.

STEP 4–BUILDING THE LEVELS OF ORGASM: Your partner might prefer going straight to an orgasm, but encourage him to build deeper levels of excitation. Begin using the tempo and pressure of licking and sucking that proves most enjoyable to him. Occasionally point his lingam towards the ground as you tightly hold the base with one hand (trapping blood in the shaft) and suck firmly on just the head.

As he approaches orgasm, (which is something he needs to communicate), slow down your stimulation and move to pleasuring other, less stimulating, areas until his arousal subsides. Pause now and again to allow the sexual energy to spread throughout his body. The more you build your partner's arousal, the more vitality he will gain from his in-jaculations and the more vitality he can share with you through his eventual ejaculation.

During the pauses, remind him to take a deep breath, stretch out his limbs, and slightly shake his arms, legs, and hips to release any pent-up energy. This will spread the ecstatic energy, release tensions, and deepen his eventual orgasms. After his arousal level has subsided, take him up and bring him down again several times until the time feels right for him to release an orgasm.

STEP 5–THE ORGASMIC RELEASE: When the ecstatic energy has filled his entire pelvic region, as well as his abdomen and thighs, it might be time to bring him through an orgasm. As he orgasms, he should use deep breaths and the tightening of his PC muscle to spread the orgasmic energy upward throughout his body. As he does so, he should focus his eyes towards the center of his forehead. This process activates the man's pineal and pituitary glands and creates a feeling of peacefulness.

When he is ready to cum, you can allow him to ejaculate in your mouth or, if you prefer, he can ejaculate on your body. If you do *not* prefer that he cum in your mouth but you *are* open to sharing advanced forms of energy exchange, then hold your partner's lingam a few inches from your face. Just before his release, visualize a ray of white light beaming forth from the tip of his lingam and into the center of your head. Continue to see and feel this energy, even as he cums and sprays onto your face or breasts.

On the other hand, if you want him to cum in your mouth, keep the lingam in your mouth as you slide in and out as deeply as possible. Simultaneously, visualize breathing light into the lingam of your partner as you make a vibration-like hum. Then, as he ejaculates, let him do so on one of your "out" movements. This allows his semen to fill your mouth and not your throat. Visualize white light being ejaculated into your mouth along with the semen, and visualize this light filling the center of your head. Once he reaches an orgasm (and ejaculates), be especially careful stimulating his lingam, particularly around the frenulum (beneath the head), as it will be highly sensitive.

STEP 6–COMING DOWN: With his semen remaining in your mouth, sit back slightly but keep your hands on his lingam and/or scrotum. Roll your eyes upwards, towards the center of your forehead and swirl the semen around in your mouth in each direction several times, thus mixing it with your saliva. At the same time, draw in several deep breaths, and contract your PC muscle with each inhalation. Release the PC contraction on each exhalation. After a few minutes, slowly swallow the juicy elixir in three parts, as you visualize a ball of light going down your throat with each gulp.

Remain still and quiet as you tune in to subtle sensations in the center of your brain and abdomen. You may feel a soft buzzing in your head and/ or a warmth or subtle vibration in your hara (navel center). Encourage your lover to become aware of waves of energy streaming through his body. Place one hand over his lingam (palm down) and the other hand over his heart, while channeling energy, love, and appreciation into these two centers of your partner. After the oral pleasuring is complete, take a soft, warm towel and gently wash every part of your partner's genitals. When the orgasm has slightly subsided, you can move to de-tumescing, or you can continue with other forms of pleasuring.

IMPORTANT REMINDERS
FOR ORALLY PLEASURING A MAN

- Orally pleasuring the penis can be combined with manually pleasuring the scrotum or prostate.

- The preferred oral technique varies from one man to another. Be sure to ask what he likes and learn by observation.

- When you notice your partner reaching the point of orgasm, unless you want him to cum, be sure to alter your stimulation to something less arousing until his urge subsides.

- Use moans and gentle body movements to let him know how great you feel when you are pleasuring him.

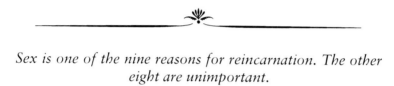

Sex is one of the nine reasons for reincarnation. The other eight are unimportant.

–Henry Miller

PART V

Intercourse

The Dance of the Divine

Most of the information prior to this section of the book could be applied individually *or* shared with a partner. This section, however, introduces concepts for those who want to learn about applying sacred sexuality in relationships with others now or in the future

Once lovers have experienced the different stages of love, energy development, and passion by exploring the variations of pleasuring (presented in the previous section of this book), they might choose to move their foreplay into intercourse. Or they might choose to let the previous explorations be sufficient for the moment without moving on to actual penetration. This decision is usually agreed upon in advance but is sometimes made *during* the intimate encounter. Either way, if the choice is made to have intercourse, there are numerous exercises and techniques to enhance this experience.

As with the previously mentioned forms of intimacy and stimulation, it's essential to maintain connection and sensitivity. **Good lovers are keenly aware of their partners.** They know their partners' stages of arousal and are able to read what's going on inside of them–physically, energetically, emotionally, mentally, and spiritually. Although this may sound like a difficult task, it becomes relatively easy when lovers are sensitive and *care enough* about each other.

Praise be to God who has placed the source of man's greatest pleasure in the woman's natural parts (genitals), and woman's greatest pleasure in the natural parts (genitals) of man.

–The Perfumed Garden

When making love, forget about orgasms. Just make love. Do it slowly enough to feel each sensation and emotion. Taking your time can result in making love for longer periods, which is certainly a great way to deepen the connection in a relationship. Avoid tensing in anticipation of an approaching orgasm, and instead, relax, focus on sharing love, and meld into each other. In fact, let go of *any* goals or agendas and of all unnecessary thoughts. **"Mindless lovemaking" is far more powerful than "mindless sex."**

Nevertheless, if you get too aroused and feel as though you will lose control, don't judge yourself. Instead, relax and observe your feelings and the sensations welling up. As you do so, the energy becomes less ejaculatory and relaxes into the inner recesses of the body. The trick is to notice and catch these desires before they sweep you away.

This section includes five chapters, each of which focuses on different forms of intercourse for various purposes.

Chapter 15–teaches how to observe signs of the varying levels of arousal in your lover.

Chapter 16–describes five groups of different sexual positions.

Chapter 17–goes to the next level and offers advanced forms of intercourse and sexploration.

Chapter 18–is a specialized theme focused on sexual healing through intercourse. This chapter presents various exercises and forms of sexual touching and intercourse specifically designed to assist in healing sexual issues, traumas, inhibitions, and blocks. Even if no signs or history of sexual trauma are present, these exercises are healing, insightful, and sensuous practices for all lovers.

Chapter 19–shares ideas on the controversial topic of threesomes and group sexual ceremonies.

Remember to communicate with each other and let your partner know when it's okay for penetration. Although lovers may intuitively know when their partners are ready for intercourse, the act of occasionally asking permission is a demonstration of respect. As with being centered enough to pause or stop at a moment's notice, this act of asking also shows self-control *and* is behavior consistent with sacred sexuality. When penetration is mutually agreeable, the lover in the dominant position (usually the one on top) can tease his or her partner by rubbing the lingam along the yoni's lips and across the clitoris. **Do whatever feels right to increase arousal, moisten the yoni, and harden the lingam, while maintaining a sense of playfulness.** When first attaining penetration, move in slowly. Then, when neither lover can wait any longer, "let the games begin."

Choosing a Partner

For some people, the concept of having a choice of the person or persons with whom to share intimacy is a novel idea. Nevertheless, not only do you have a choice, but on some level, you have always been involved in creating your partners (or their manifestation into your life). As you learn and evolve, you develop and demonstrate more self-love and self-worth. You then find that your healthier, more confident state of mind has a dramatic effect on the quality of people you attract into your life and with whom you choose to share deeper intimacy.

If, on the other hand, you are already in a relationship, you probably experience one (or a combination) of the following types.

1. Your partner is on the same path and *is* willing to share concepts such as sacred sexuality.

2. Your partner is open to *limited* exploration.

3. Your partner is *not* open to exploring greater forms of true lovemaking.

The last category is unfortunately the most common and creates problems that are not easily solved. In such cases, prayer and couples counseling probably offer the most hope. If your partner is not open to either of these options, it's time to take a serious look at what you would like to experience in your life, now, and in the future. **Remember, sacred sexuality and living bliss are about experiencing the life of love, joy, purpose, and passion that God gifted you since the beginning of time, not about settling for less or bargaining your life away.**

Emotionally and spiritually mature practitioners of sacred sexuality, never have a shortage of potential lovers. There are always wonderful people with whom you can share, not necessarily sexually. Yet, in this evolving state of maturity, you are never irresponsibly promiscuous.

In sacred sexuality, the concept of *growing* relationships (from friendships to life-mates) is honored as a responsible means of assuring the most evolved partnerships. Yet, there is a point in your spiritual evolution where you can love someone immediately. This ability to share *immediate* love does not replace the value of growing a relationship over time. Nevertheless, there comes a stage in development where the true love of the soul can be shared with anyone, at any time, and in any form.

When sharing sacred sexuality, there are several different types of relationships from which to choose. They are as follows:

1. **Mutual Using**–occurs when two mature, emotionally healthy, consenting adults agree that they will share sexually; yet they are merely borrowing each other momentarily (and with no attachments) for the purpose of the experience. This is commonly referred to as "mutual usery." They are not necessarily friends, but they are choosing to be lovers (once or a hundred times). Again, there are no attachments or agendas.

2. **Intimate Friendships**–are relationships that have all the traits of a good friendship, such as honesty, good communication, playfulness, and longevity. However, the friends involved have decided to trust each other with occasional intimacy as well, which can take many forms, ranging from holding each other to full-on sexual intercourse.

3. **Monogamous Partnering**–is, of course, the committed, intimate relationship between two people. The partners have agreed to be faithful to each other. They may be trying out such an arrangement on a short-term basis or they may be life-mates.

4. **Multiple Partners**–is best practiced by only the most responsible individuals. Having more than one lover can easily be an unconscious cover for issues ranging from a lack of commitment to sexual addiction. Therefore, people who choose this experience need to undergo a thorough self-inventory to understand their motivations and assure they are honorable. People with numerous lovers must be honest with themselves and all other parties concerned about their choice of lifestyle. A person with multiple lovers must also practice the safest sex possible.

5. **The Sacred Sexual Relationship**–exists only in theory. There is no exact definition because it varies greatly from person to person and couple to couple. Furthermore, a sacred sexual relationship can apply in any of the above definitions, as well as a combination of most of the above.

CHAPTER 15

Signs of the Times

Reading Your Lover's Response

Taoist sexologists teach that there are five signs to observe to see if a woman is aroused enough for intercourse. In *Secret Methods: Sexual Recipes of the Plain Girl*, Taoist masters offer thorough instructions on how a couple should prepare for intercourse. Heeding the advice of these instructions assists lovers in developing a greater understanding of their partners' states of arousal–an essential awareness in sacred sexuality. Furthermore, such practices encourage greater sensitivity between lovers concerning their needs, fluctuations in energy levels, and the gradual buildup of sexual energy.

If you don't know the way of intercourse, partaking of herbs {aphrodisiacs} is of no benefit.

–P'eng Tsu

Essentially, the first steps are to achieve the *moistening of the yoni* and *hardening of the lingam*, demonstrating the healthy presence of the *yin* and *yang* principles. Then, it is essential for the man to observe several signs to determine whether or not his partner is prepared for intercourse–to know her stage of arousal and, consequently, what to do next. These signals are known as *The Five Signs, The Five Desires*, and *The Ten Stages of Loving*.

The first of these signals are *The Five Signs* that describe the involuntary sexual responses of an aroused woman. They are as follows:

1. Reddened face and chest
2. Hard nipples and beads of sweat
3. Parched throat
4. Dry lips
5. Moistening in the yoni

The Five Desires depict the levels of response in a woman's body. Through careful observation and very little verbal communication, her lover can know exactly where she is in her stages of ecstasy and, as a result, adjust his technique to meet her needs.

1. The first desire–intent–is demonstrated by a quick pulse and shallow breath.
2. The second desire–awareness–is demonstrated with flared nostrils and parted lips.
3. The third desire–the peak of passion–is demonstrated by the building, rhythmic movements of her body.
4. The fourth desire–concentration–is demonstrated by a warm sweat, which manifests during the initial stages of her orgasm.
5. The fifth desire–an ecstatic orgasm–occurs when her eyes close, her body tenses, and then releases.

Finally, there are *The Ten Stages of Loving,* which are signs that a man is wise to observe. Through the movements of her body, a woman communicates to her lover what she would like him to do.

1. The woman embraces her lover, which means she wants to feel his lingam against her.
2. The woman stretches out and arches bringing attention to her yoni, which means she wants it pleasured.
3. The woman stretches her legs and mid-section, which means she wants penetration.
4. The woman shakes and rocks her pelvis, which means she is feeling great pleasure.
5. The woman raises her legs and grabs her lover with her feet, which means she does not want him to move away.
6. The woman squeezes her thighs together, which means she wants to feel the lingam as much as possible.

7. The woman moves her body rhythmically from side to side, which means she would like vigorous thrusting from different angles.

8. The woman presses her upper body and breasts against her beloved or pulls him close, which means she is nearing orgasm.

9. The woman relaxes as if she has left her body, which means that waves of pleasure are moving through her.

10. The woman's vital juices (*amrita*) are released from her yoni, which means she is fully satisfied.

THE NINE FEMALE ATTAINMENTS

A humorous metaphor for the sexual encounter of a man and woman states that to attend to a woman's needs, a man must learn to get her water boiling before he puts in his vegetables (lingam); otherwise, the vegetables may become soggy or limp. Besides the aforementioned observations that reveal when and how a woman wants to be touched, Taoists also suggest nine stages of arousal to look for in a woman to know if her water is boiling and to assure that she is fully charged with sexual energy. The first four are the most common and are reached by most women. With sufficient foreplay and arousal, a woman's body attains the following four levels:

1. Energy fills the lungs when she begins to breathe rapidly and salivate.

2. Energy fills the heart when she extends her tongue and begins to kiss passionately.

3. Energy fills the spleen, pancreas, and stomach when she begins to hug tightly.

4. Energy fills the kidneys and genitals when she grows moist and experiences basic vaginal contractions or orgasms.

At this point, if her partner maintains a steady stimulation, preferably without altering the pace or contact, a woman's body reaches new levels of arousal. She feels a fuller awakening as she moves more freely until she loses control and surrenders to a fuller, total-being orgasm. The Taoists describe these extra five stages as follows:

5. Energy fills the bones and joints when she moves her pelvis and bites gently.

6. Energy fills the liver when she presses against her partner and wraps around him.

7. Energy fills the blood when she rubs her partner and caresses his penis.

8. Energy fills the muscles when her body relaxes.

9. Energy fills the entire body when she moans in ecstasy and surrenders.

THE FOUR ATTAINMENTS OF THE "JADE STALK"

Taoists also describe a man's stages of sexual arousal and excitement. His partner is advised to assist him in reaching all four levels, as his fully charged lingam (which Taoists refer to as the "Jade Stalk") also assures *her* of the greatest pleasure. Although most of these four stages should be reached *before* making love, it *is* possible for many of them to be attained *after* penetrating the yoni, or "sacred space."

1. *Firmness* is the first attainment and shows that sexual energy has filled his yin and yang aspects.

2. *Swelling* is the second attainment and shows that sexual energy has filled his blood.

3. *Hardness* is the third attainment and shows that sexual energy has filled his bones.

4. *Heat* is the fourth attainment and shows that sexual energy has filled his spirit.

If lovers observe and respond to the majority of these signs of arousal, they will increase their sensitivity and lovemaking skills. Pursuing and encouraging these stages also builds more intense levels of arousal and readiness for intercourse, resulting in a more intense total-being, orgasmic response.

CHAPTER 16

Sexual Positions

Five Sets of Positions

Once lovers have decided to share intercourse, they can let nature takes its course and gradually discover which positions feel best to them. Or they can playfully explore the various positions defined by the arts of sacred sexuality. In either case, the movement from one position to another should be as fluid, effortless, and natural as possible.

Although sacred sexual practices are not about performing sexual calisthenics and having intercourse in as many positions as possible, it *is* advisable to playfully explore several positions during most of your lovemaking experiences. Every system of sacred sexuality has numerous suggested positions for lovemaking. For the purpose of simplicity, they are grouped here into five basic sets: man on top, woman on top, lying on sides, man from behind, and miscellaneous. The last category includes positions that do not fit into the first four groups: for example, when neither person is "on top" (such as standing positions) nor are they both "lying on their sides" (such as when both lovers lie on their backs).

Be sure to see beyond the sexual anatomy of your lover and the stimulation of the genitals. Instead, gradually expand your focus to an awareness of the entire person. Imagine feeling ecstatic energy flowing throughout *your* body and the body of your lover.

Once again, sexual positions are essentially yoga postures adapted to a specific form of practice. These positions are good for the health and healing of both partners and are effective for creating energy circuits between lovers. The different angles of penetration stimulate healing to various parts of the body, including organs and glands. Furthermore, the variations, when done with intensity and passion, become an effective cardiovascular exercise.

Or, when done slowly and tenderly, they provide numerous opportunities for creating a deeper, soul-level connection between lovers.

MAN ON TOP

Despite its reputation for being the most conservative sexual position, the missionary position (man on top) is the best position for aligning genitals and hearts, as well as allowing a face-to-face connection. This position permits the maximum amount of skin contact, while enabling continued kissing.

The missionary position is also one of the most natural and comfortable positions and exerts the least effort on the part of both lovers. As with all of the major sets of positions, the man-on-top has several variations. These variations are easily explored by experimenting with leg positions, each of which offers completely different sensations. For example, by placing the woman's knees against her chest (with feet up on his shoulders) the man achieves deeper penetration and has the option of viewing his lingam as he does so.

This position should be avoided by pregnant women and by couples where the man is excessively heavy.

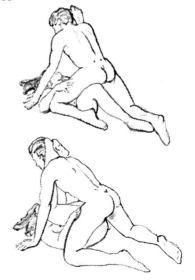

VARIATIONS INCLUDE:

1. Missionary with leg variations
2. Knees up–feet to chest or over shoulders
3. Her legs wrapped around his hips
4. Her pelvis elevated

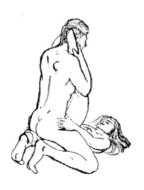

WOMAN ON TOP

When the woman is in the position of sexual control (being on top), wonderful things can happen. First of all, she can control her arousal level and overall preferences as to the tempo and depth of penetration. This set of positions allows for maximum stimulation to the clitoris, which usually doesn't make contact with a thrusting lingam. For these reasons, the woman-on-top positions are the second most popular in lovemaking.

In the woman-on-top positions, the woman can sit facing or turned away from her lover, or she can lie on top of him. She can also sit in a squatting position, which adds incredible stimulation to his lingam.

The most difficult aspect of the women-on-top positions is that some of them require much physical work and endurance, especially for the woman's thighs–which may be why she usually lets her lover be on top. But a woman can strengthen her thighs and build her endurance by practicing squatting exercises. She can also exercise by getting down on her hands and knees with her elbows on the floor and thrusting her pelvis back and forth for three to five minutes.

VARIATIONS INCLUDE:

1. She sits facing him
2. She sits facing the opposite direction
3. She sits in a squatting position
4. She lies on him in various missionary positions

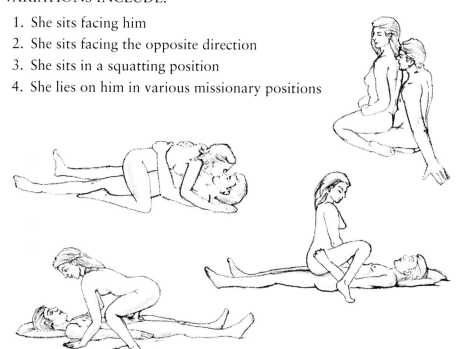

LYING ON SIDES

This set of positions includes the ever-popular and very intimate position of "spooning," wherein the man lies behind the woman, while both of them are lying on their sides. This position gives a snuggling feeling and provides whole-body contact.

When lying on their sides, the man can also lie at a right angle to the woman (either facing her back or her front), as well as experimenting with the variations of holding one of her legs up in the air.

The drawback to any position where both partners are on their sides is that the man might find it a challenge to achieve just the right angle for penetration.

VARIATIONS INCLUDE:

1. Both partners lie on their sides and face each other
2. She faces him with legs wrapped around him
3. He suspends one of her legs
4. They both lie on their sides with her back to him in the "spooning" position

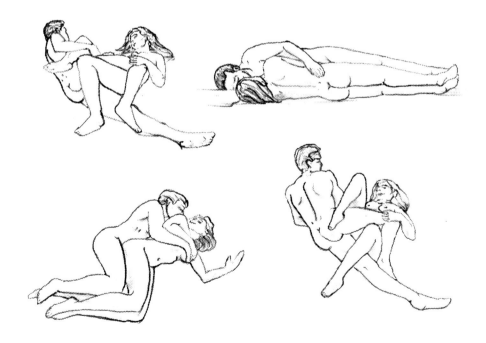

MAN FROM BEHIND

The variations of man-from-behind positions include the woman bending over a bed (or similar object) or bending forward on her hands and knees (doggy style) or bending from the waist down with her hands toward the floor. Whichever the choice, these positions are often convenient for the woman to reach under and stimulate her clitoris and/or fondle the man's genitals.

Some couples find this set of positions to be the best for G-spot access. Also, they are very primal positions, so the man often feels powerful as he grips the woman's waist from behind and thrusts in and out.

The down side of the man-from-behind position is that it can seem somewhat impersonal. Also, it's easy for the man to accidentally penetrate too far into the woman's yoni. So caution should be taken.

VARIATIONS INCLUDE:

1. Animal style
2. She is bent forward
3. She lies flat with him lying on her back

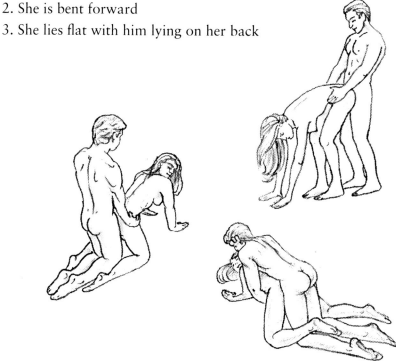

MISCELLANEOUS POSITIONS

The following set of sexual positions is the most diverse because it includes any position that doesn't fall under one of the previously mentioned sets. These miscellaneous positions include such variations as standing (the male is facing his partner but is not technically "on top"), both partners lying back, and both partners sitting and facing each other (with the woman on the man's lap).

Most people will agree that having sex in various standing positions is thought to be (and portrayed in movies as) highly erotic. Standing positions work well for tight spaces such as showers, for "quickies," and for passionate moments when the mood is so "hot" you can't wait to find a more comfortable location. Standing variations also stimulate a sense of daring and exhibitionism.

However, the disadvantages of standing positions are many. First of all, they are the most physically challenging for the male, as he usually has one hand propping up his partner's leg or her whole body. It's also difficult for his lingam to angle up and underneath his partner for penetration. Furthermore, it's hard for either partner to use their hands for additional stimulation.

VARIATIONS INCLUDE:

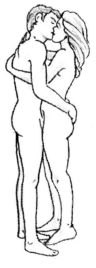

1. Standing
2. Woman suspended
3. She lies back but he sits up
4. She lies back and he lies back
5. The couple sits facing each other

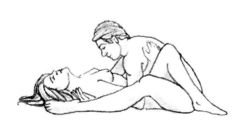

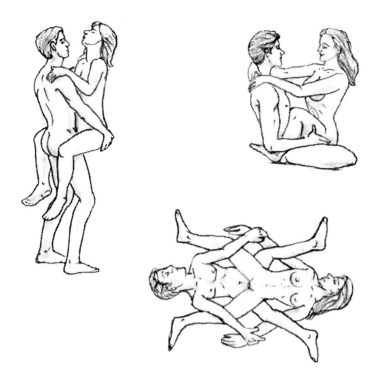

CHAPTER 17

Enhancing Intercourse

Sexploration

When a couple chooses to expand their knowledge and repertoire of lovemaking and intercourse, they should consider learning more advanced techniques and positions. This learning can include specific uses of thrusts and movements.

The following techniques are varied in their intents and purposes. Some primarily assist the male, while others assist the female. Nevertheless, any chosen technique will add to the pleasure of both partners and, in the long run, bring healing to them–individually and as a couple. After finding an exercise that works well, repeat it as often as you like or move on to other playful experiences.

VARIOUS THRUSTS FOR THE MALE

By practicing various forms of thrusting, a man can learn what his partner enjoys the most. Also, by varying his thrusts, he can maintain his erection for a longer period, since the pauses during the alterations allow his arousal to subside–even if only slightly. The following are variations of thrusts of the lingam:

1. **Back and Forth**–The lingam slowly glides back and forth in the standard lovemaking fashion.
2. **Churning**–The lingam is held in the man's hand and the head is churned inside the yoni.
3. **Upper Rubbing**–The lingam is angled to stimulate the G-spot during thrusts.
4. **Lower Rubbing**–The lingam is angled to stimulate the lower part of the yoni's opening during thrusts.

5. **Short Thrusts**–The lingam is withdrawn only halfway and then thrust in again.

6. **Long Thrusts**–The lingam is withdrawn completely and then thrust inside.

7. **Thrusting Hard**–This can be done with short or long thrusts but is done as hard as is comfortable for both partners.

8. **Pressing**–The lingam carefully penetrates as far as possible and then is made to swell or enlarge slightly.

THREE DEPTHS OF THRUSTING

Although not commonly known, there are three depths of penetration that can be achieved by the male. Each level, or depth, of thrusting is invaluable for different reasons. A shallow thrust, for example, can be used by the male to tease his lover and heighten arousal. On the other hand, a semi-full depth can be helpful for a couple who experience pain or discomfort with full-depth penetration, usually from the length of his lingam or shortness of her yoni's depth. Finally, the full-depth penetration can be used either for extra stimulation when the sexual organs are compatible or to add extension for a male whose lingam is shorter than his lover's yoni.

1. **Shallow Depth**–The male uses his thighs to avoid complete entry.

2. **Semi-full Depth**–The male enters until his pubic bone reaches his partner and is flush with his thighs.

3. **Full-depth**–The male enters all the way, shifts both pelvic bones outward, which allows the sacrum to thrust the lingam forward. This thrust should be done carefully and only with his partner's permission.

VARIOUS THRUSTS FOR THE FEMALE

When the woman takes control of intercourse, she can experience a wonderful sense of empowerment and confidence. Although she may have to push through inhibitions, self-criticism, and perhaps even a lack of muscle strength, the results are well worth it. When she chooses to take control, she must understand the responsibilities that go along with being in the "driver's seat." In other words, she must know when she is moving *too quickly* or *too slowly* because her partner can lose his erection either from *too much* stimulation (resulting in a premature orgasm) or from *not enough* stimulation (resulting in a loss of arousal).

Each of the "female-superior" positions presents challenges to a woman's coordination and strength, especially in her leg muscles. Additionally, each variation offers a unique form of stimulation for her and her lover. Therefore, she should take time to explore all positions.

1. **Gliding**–The woman sits on her lover's lingam while facing him. She places her hands down on either side of his head with her breasts over his face and begins rocking her body back and forth as his lingam slides in and out of her yoni.

2. **Pelvic Rocking**–The woman inserts her lover's lingam as deeply as she likes and then begins rocking her pelvis back and forth with her clitoris rubbing against his pubic bone.

3. **Pelvic Rotating**–This is similar to pelvic rocking, but instead of rocking back and forth, the woman makes circles with her pelvis.

4. **Backing In**–The woman faces away from her lover while on her knees and backs in, sliding herself onto his lingam and then begins thrusting. This is similar to gliding but facing the opposite direction.

5. **Squatting**–The woman inserts her lover's lingam as she sits on him in a squatting position. Her hands are usually placed on the floor for support, but her knees are kept off the floor. Her feet are usually flat on the floor, and her hips are kept suspended, not sitting in a resting position. In this position, she carefully slides down his lingam and then lifts again and continues down and up.

Variations of Intercourse

If you choose to, you can expand upon your repertoire of intercourse positions by experimenting with such variations as those found below. Most of the choices found in this set of variations are *passive* forms of lovemaking. These positions focus less on developing *physical sensations* and, instead, focus on increasing your awareness of the *energy* between you and your lover. These are *crucial* options for your repertoire, as they are some of the best forms of intercourse for developing trust and intimacy.

TECHNIQUE:
Energetic Intercourse

Men and women have grown accustomed to thinking that intercourse must involve genital penetration. Consequently, it is crucial for lovers

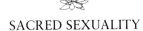
to practice such higher levels of sharing as energetic lovemaking. It's a delightful variation of lovemaking. Once this technique becomes familiar, lovers can incorporate it into any form of sexual encounter or have moments of sharing only energetic intercourse.

STEP 1: Sit comfortably with the woman on the man's lap. Practice some form of connecting (such as dedicated prayer, words of love and respect or toning).

STEP 2: Begin sending energy to each other's genitals. As you exhale (and your partner inhales), lightly press out your perineum, and send a wave of light to your partner's genitals. As you inhale (and your partner exhales), lightly contract your perineum and imagine that you are drawing your partner's genitals towards you.

STEP 3: As you inhale, simultaneously become aware of your heart center filling with love. On your exhale, channel that love through your genitals and to your partner, while your partner simultaneously inhales. Begin feeling a greater sense of oneness.

STEP 4: Now, when you send your genital energy to your partner on your exhale (and your partner's inhale), send it into his or her genitals and up the spine to the top of the head. Repeat this several times.

STEP 5: When the time feels right, make a connection with your mouths and tongues. After you send your next surge of energy into your partner's genitals and up his or her spine, on your next inhale draw the energy you sent into your lover, out of his or her mouth and into your heart. On the next exhale, again send energy down through your genitals and into your partner's genitals. Repeat this circulation several times.

STEP 6: Allow yourselves to meld into the kisses and energy circulation. If the genitals are aroused and the pelvises are gyrating or if an orgasm occurs, let it happen. However, the primary goal is to remain focused on the energetic exchange.

STEP 7: After practicing this lovemaking technique for twenty to thirty minutes (or more), gradually draw your attention and breath back into your own body. Become aware of your pulse and any energy surges. Slowly separate your bodies and begin stretching. After several minutes of silent integration, join for a hug of gratitude and take time to share feedback.

TECHNIQUE:
The Next Step

The following technique is similar to the "energetic intercourse" exercise, except there is actual genital penetration. This technique is a good bridge between the physical and energetic forms of intercourse because it combines the two. It is especially effective for those partners who have difficulty feeling the energy exchange in the "energetic intercourse" technique. It's also a great intercourse technique for healing sexual trauma.

STEP 1: Remove all clothing and sit comfortably with the woman on the man's lap. Practice some form of connecting (such as a dedicated prayer, words of love and respect or toning).

STEP 2: Begin sending energy to each other's genitals. As you exhale (and your partner inhales), lightly press out your perineum and send a wave of light to your partner's genitals. As you inhale (and your partner exhales), lightly contract your perineum and imagine that you are drawing your partner's genitals towards you.

STEP 3: As you inhale, simultaneously become aware of your heart centers filling with love. On your exhale, channel that love through your genitals and to your partner, while your partner simultaneously inhales. Begin feeling a greater sense of oneness.

STEP 4: Both partners place one hand on their lover's heart, while the other hand strokes their lover's genitals as they both moan and move in a way that creates arousal.

STEP 5: When the time feels right, the woman sits up slightly and inserts her partner's lingam. If it is needed, she can assist with some lubricant.

STEP 6: The woman then begins moving her pelvis and rocks back and forth to create greater arousal. The male should warn his partner if he gets too stimulated and is approaching an orgasm. If this occurs, she can pause, run her fingers upwards along his spine, drawing the orgasmic energy away from the genitals. Once the orgasmic sensation has passed, she can begin moving again.

STEP 7: The man should refrain from having an orgasm for as long as possible. Then, perhaps when his partner reaches a climax, the two lovers can release at the same time. When orgasm occurs, the partners should allow the release of ecstatic moans, while simultaneously shaking their bodies as they cum. This release of sound and movement assists in the distribution of ecstatic energy throughout the body.

STEP 8: Finally, gradually draw your attention and breath back into your own body. Become aware of your pulse and any energy surges. After several minutes of silent integration, spend time embracing in gratitude and take time to share feedback.

TECHNIQUE:
Full-Body Connecting

The following technique is similar to "energetic intercourse" but involves more intimate contact. This exercise can be done in a sitting position (with the woman on the man's lap) or in the lying position as described below.

STEP 1: The female partner lies comfortably on her back with her knees bent and open and with her partner lying on top of her.

STEP 2: She wraps her arms and legs around him and hooks her feet together, creating a feeling of total body connection.

STEP 3: After a moment of joining, she inserts his lingam into her yoni and begins gently connecting mouths with deep, tender kisses. Pause occasionally to exchange glances, sighs, and moans.

STEP 4: Be aware of your entire body melding into your partner's.

STEP 5: The male should occasionally move his pelvis enough to maintain an erection and then return to a still, centered presence. If the mind drifts at any time during this exercise, draw it back to the present moment.

TECHNIQUE:
Yab Yum (Male-Female Union)

Yab means "male principle," and *yum* means "female principle." Therefore, the *yab yum* position represents a union of the cosmic male and female dualities. This is a wonderful, passive position for making love or simply connecting. The *yab yum* position can be practiced with the couple having intercourse and closely interlocking bodies, arms, legs, mouths, and genitals. It can also be performed more passively with the couple sitting together, yet keeping their torsos slightly separated to enable them to gaze into each other's eyes, as well as share loving comments.

STEP 1: Mutually decide whether or not this position will at any time include insertion of the lingam.

STEP 2: Sit apart from each other. Say a brief prayer, asking to feel love and interconnectedness.

STEP 3: Then the woman sits on the man's lap and wraps her legs around him.

STEP 4: Lean slightly back and gaze into each other's eyes as you breathe gently. Meld into each other's energy for an indefinite period of time.

STEP 5: When the time is right, express your feelings for each other. Even if this level of intimacy evokes laughter or crying, continue the sharing.

STEP 6: After the verbal sharing, rest your heads on each other's shoulders. Breathe together and share feelings of deep gratitude.

STEP 7: When you are finished, take time to stretch and do grounding exercises.

TECHNIQUE:

Yin-Style Sex

Yin-style lovemaking is only for those partners who are prepared to spend time joining as one with no other sexual agendas. The partners will spend at least thirty minutes in a state of totally passive intercourse without physical orgasms. The focus will be on connecting and relaxing completely into the experience of each other's energy.

Yin-style intercourse challenges priorities because with this technique, love must be the primary focus, as it should be in all lovemaking. However, in most forms of intercourse, movement of the bodies and excessive stimulation often distract the participants from the awareness of love.

Yin-style sex involves floating in a relaxed state of loving euphoria before, during, and after intercourse. This passive state activates the parasympathetic nervous system and is distinctly different from the usual biological forms of intense, goal-oriented sex that activate the sympathetic nervous system with its "fight or flight" response.

STEP 1: Prayerfully state to your partner what you most wish to experience in your time together.

STEP 2: Sit in the *yab yum* position with the woman on the man's lap.

STEP 3: After inserting the man's lingam, embrace each other and sit very still. Do not move your bodies, pelvises, or genitals until the lingam needs restimulating to maintain an erection.

STEP 4: Keep your minds empty of all thoughts. Feel deeply into your soul and the soul of your partner.

STEP 5: When it's time to conclude, hug and thank each other for the wonderful sharing.

TECHNIQUE:
Intercourse Practicing In-jaculation

The general purpose for using in-jaculation as a solo exercise or as a technique during intercourse is to channel sexual energy upward through the body. In so doing, the energy moves along the central acupuncture meridian (which feeds all the major organ meridians) as well as through the spine, thus feeding the central nervous system. The in-jaculation process takes the man's sexual energy that is usually wasted through shallow sex and pelvic ejaculations and turns his sexual force into creative energy for self-empowerment and rejuvenation, improving overall health and vitality.

STEP 1: Before making love, decide on a signal word to use when it's time to pause all stimulation.

STEP 2: During intercourse, when arousal reaches a moment just prior to the point of no return, use your signal word to notify your partner that you need to pause all stimulation.

STEP 3: During the pause, your partner can assist your in-jaculation by stroking her hand along your spine in an upward motion, while visualizing the movement of energy in that same direction.

STEP 4: Also during the pause, place your tongue on the roof of your mouth, begin inhaling deeply through your nose and exhaling through your mouth, while simultaneously contracting your Kegel/PC muscle on the inhale and visualizing the energy moving up to the top of your head.

STEP 5: Then, as you exhale, allow the energy to flow down the front of your body, past your heart center, and into your navel center (which is located approximately two to three inches below your navel). Visualize the energy swirling in your naval center, where it will be stored for the body's future use as vitality.

STEP 6: Repeat this in-jaculation cycle at least three times before proceeding with lovemaking.

CHAPTER 18

Intercourse for Healing

Sexual Healing Techniques

All trauma seeks a home or hideout somewhere in the body. When it does so, it wraps itself in muscle tissue and makes itself cozy–hoping never to be found, which is unlikely since it will inevitably cause discomfort. These same traumas also get lodged in the body in other ways. For example, the *energy* of the **trauma stores in the *energy field,* while *emotions* related to such trauma store in the *emotional body.*** In any case, something painful and foreign to the body and soul gets locked in. Sometimes these hurts begin to fester. Other times, they tend to go numb. Still other times the pain remains completely present and tender to the touch. Finally, at other times, the pain remains present but places muscular armor around itself. In such circumstances, the armor can be lovingly touched and gradually broken down. Of course, this means that eventually there can be a sudden awakening of pain in the tissue. When this occurs during a sexual healing massage, back off slightly and rub gently, vibrate your finger or hold it completely still until it feels appropriate to move in again for more healing massage, which sometimes has to wait for another day.

Many individuals have sexual inhibitions or dysfunctions that include difficulty reaching an orgasm through intercourse alone. Sacred sexuality can be useful for healing such issues. **Although sexual healing may not be the primary focus of the sexual experience, sexual issues of repression or trauma can be brought to the lovemaking session and patiently addressed.**

All such repressed or stored trauma can have an effect on a person's health and sexuality. **The aftermath of sexual trauma can impact the psyche**

in such a way that it prevents a person from letting go and experiencing true orgasm. Stored trauma also results in a lack of trust, and of course, this absence of trust makes the experience of sacred sexuality impossible.

The more often a woman has intercourse without taking the time to go through her natural stages of arousal and preparation, the thicker the tissue within her yoni becomes, thus decreasing her sensitivity. Furthermore, when she moves her pelvis too much, she unconsciously tightens her pelvic and vaginal muscles, which, once again, creates an unhealthy patterning in her sexual anatomy. Ironically, a woman may think she is sexually healthy and responsive to stimulation, but sometimes her arousal does not result from sexual health and vitality. Rather, it results from her sexual anatomy becoming hardened and giving off false signs of arousal.

The male lingam can also become traumatized from physical and sexual abuse, as well as from excessive masturbation. For example, if a man gets used to quick ejaculations from fast-paced masturbation, he can become premature in his ejaculations. Excessive masturbation might also make his lingam numb to pleasuring by a partner.

The release of repressed pain from trauma often results in the ability to experience deeper forms of orgasm. For example, after releasing stored trauma, a person will feel an increase in energetic orgasms or perhaps emotional orgasms. However, it is not wise to *expect* such results, especially when sexual touching is for healing purposes.

When purposely applying healing touch to the genitals, be sure to include the elements of love and playfulness. Be sure to sanitize, play soothing music, and keep lubricants nearby. Place a trashcan close-by to discard used tissue or in case the person receiving the healing gets nauseous, which is rare, but possible, with such deep emotional work.

When you give healing massage to the genitals or an adjacent region, remind your partner to breathe deeply. While you are massaging, don't be surprised if you discover points of discomfort. As you hold and rub these tender regions, make sure to remain connected with your partner. Avoid sudden movements that may startle or harm your partner. Instead, move slowly.

TECHNIQUE:

Reconnecting the Numb Parts

Once again, trauma and personal issues can cause the body's sensual organs and responses to become inhibited or even shut down. Although this process usually occurs in the erogenous zones, it can occur in any part of the body. Various forms of reconnective healing can reawaken the body and reverse the effects of trauma. The following is an exercise designed to heal and reawaken "frozen" areas of the body:

STEP 1: Choose the most easily "turned-on" part of your body.

STEP 2: Begin stimulating this area until it is aroused.

STEP 3: Now choose the region of your body that seems to be inhibited or shut down.

STEP 4: Begin stimulating this area in the same manner (tempo and pressure) you are stimulating the easily "turned-on" region.

STEP 5: After both areas have been stimulated, begin alternating from one to the other. Try adding energy massage techniques to stimulate the areas, making whatever body part that needs healing reach out for you. To reach out, it has to wake up.

TECHNIQUE:

G-spot Massage

The primary purpose for yoni (vaginal) and G-spot massage is to access and release any unhealthy feelings or cellular memories resulting from sexual trauma. Remember, sexual trauma can take the form of rape, molestation or shaming from others. Sexual trauma can also result from having sex without a loving connection with the other person involved. Cellular memories of such events are stored in the body's tissue and, if left unhealed, affect a person's health, vitality, and sexual response. Yoni massage is one of the best methods of releasing such trauma. A woman can do this massage for herself, or she can have a partner, friend or properly trained healer assist her. Whoever is chosen, it must be understood that yoni healing massage should not be done in conjunction with or prior to intercourse. The traumatized cells within the yoni need time to rest and reprogram. Therefore, the time after healing work is best spent meditating and connecting.

STEP 1: Sit comfortably facing each other and synchronize your breathing.

Look into each other's eyes. When a connection is felt, share a prayer for healing. Have a fresh supply of tissue nearby in case of tears. Also, play soothing music–something she likes.

STEP 2: The woman receiving the yoni massage should lie comfortably on her back. Because of the sensitivity of this healing, it is essential that she is comfortable and supported by plenty of pillows.

STEP 3: As the two of you continue taking deep centering breaths, place one hand on the woman's heart-center and the other hand gently and carefully over her pubic bone.

STEP 4: After a few minutes, gently begin moving your hands back and forth across her body, giving her a light massage. Afterwards, reconnect with your partner's heart and pubic region.

STEP 5: Lubricate your massaging hand thoroughly and warm the oil before you make contact with the woman's skin. Then place this hand over her yoni and hold for a minute. Rest your other hand on the woman's lower abdomen as support.

STEP 6: Gradually begin moving your massaging hand and gently lubricating the entire yoni. Once the yoni is evenly lubricated, take more time to specifically massage each section. Begin with the outer lips, then move on to the minor lips. Keep in mind, this contact is not meant to stimulate arousal; it's meant to lubricate the yoni and to gain trust.

STEP 7: When the time is right, ask permission to move your finger(s) to the inside of the yoni. Once you do so, take time to massage all of the walls of the vagina. Begin with the two side walls. Move to massaging the floor of the vagina, which is in the direction of the spine and colon.

STEP 8: Then rotate your hand so that your palm faces the pubic bone. From this position, begin massaging the G-spot and surrounding region. Be sure to give attention to *all* the parts of the yoni. As you contact areas that are either numb or painful, be extra careful and sensitive. Gently massage the tender spots or just hold your finger there for a minute. As you do so, send prayerful and loving thoughts into the spot being healed.

STEP 9: After the tender area releases some of its tension, move on to other areas until all areas have been worked on and the healing massage feels complete. In the event that an area does not release and begin to feel less tenderness, just gently touch it and hold still with prayerful intent. Then move on. You may have to return to this spot at a later date.

STEP 10: When the massaging is concluded, hold one hand over the yoni and another over the heart while visualizing an energy connection between these two areas.

STEP 11: Spend several minutes meditating together. Ask the woman receiving the healing to visualize a soft white light filling her body and caressing every inch of her yoni.

STEP 12: For the next few minutes, when she inhales, she should focus on the words "love and safety." Then, with each exhale, she should focus on the words "And so it is."

STEP 13: When concluded, do some grounding and stretching. Getting fresh air is also highly advisable.

TECHNIQUE:
The Healing Lingam

Despite its reputation as a symbol of aggression, when used properly, the lingam is one of the best tools for sexual healing. The following technique is particularly useful when a woman has a history of pain or tenderness during intercourse or finger penetration.

STEP 1: The woman lies back in an effortless, comfortable position. She should feel as though she is floating on a cloud.

STEP 2: Her partner (or healer) uses plenty of lubrication to assist his lingam in effortlessly penetrating her yoni.

STEP 3: His penetration is slow and gentle, not thrusting.

STEP 4: The woman remains highly aware of her body to sense any physical discomforts within her yoni.

STEP 5: If a tender area is found, her partner holds completely still against the tender spot (for just a moment), and then backs off slightly, allowing enough space to create a healing vortex within the yoni. Simultaneously, the couple gazes lovingly into each other's eyes.

STEP 6: Both partners visualize a soft blue or white light gently swirling in the space between the lingam and yoni. Soon, the woman should feel a release of the tenderness. If not, repeat this exercise a few times. If the tenderness still does not release, be patient. Move onto other exercises that are more comfortable, and try this technique at a later time.

TECHNIQUE:
Ten Sets of Nine

The "Sets-of-Nine" exercise is a well-known Taoist technique designed to aid in developing concentration and maintaining an erection. To prepare, make sure both partners are in comfortable positions where the male can easily control the depth of his thrusts. Then, the male slides his lingam into the woman's yoni with varying deep and shallow thrusts but always totaling ten with each set. Altogether there are nine sets of ten strokes, which are practiced as follows:

STEP 1: Insert only the head of the lingam into the yoni. Then withdraw (the first shallow stroke). Repeat these shallow strokes nine times total, and then on the tenth stroke, carefully thrust the entire lingam into the yoni at once (the first deep stroke).

STEP 2: Follow with eight shallow strokes (only head of lingam) and two deep strokes (entire lingam).

STEP 3: Do seven shallow and three deep strokes.

STEP 4: Do six shallow and four deep strokes.

STEP 5: Do five shallow and five deep strokes.

STEP 6: Do four shallow and six deep strokes.

STEP 7: Do three shallow and seven deep strokes.

STEP 8: Do two shallow and eight deep strokes.

STEP 9: Finally, do one shallow followed by nine deep strokes.

TECHNIQUE:
Intercourse with a Limp Penis

The advantages of occasionally making love with a limp penis (lingam) are numerous. First of all, it prepares both partners for moments when the male may not be able to achieve an erection. It also helps to remove the belief that the penis must be erect for the man to make love or as a symbol of successful lovemaking. Having intercourse with a limp penis allows a unique, yin-like softness to be shared between the penis and yoni. It's especially helpful if the man's penis is too large or uncomfortable to insert when fully erect.

STEP 1: Find the most comfortable position possible to give you easy access for inserting the penis.

STEP 2: Either partner should clasp the penis with two fingers, just below the head and guide it into the yoni.

STEP 3: Once the head of the penis is inserted, move the two-finger clasp to the middle of the penis and guide it in further.

STEP 4: Now move the two-finger clasp to the base of the penis and once again guide the penis in.

STEP 5: Hold each other closely and comfortably. The woman must practice non-tensing of her yoni or else her vaginal muscles will force out the man's penis.

STEP 6: Move the pelvis occasionally to keep the penis firm enough to stay inside. Otherwise, remain motionless and absorb each other's energy and essence. You might experiment with going to sleep in this position.

Assisting Orgasms

If there are continuing problems with your partner reaching orgasm during intercourse, it can mean his or her genitals need awakening.

In that case, it helps to see your partner as a man or woman whose orgasm is like a shyness or inhibition that needs to be patiently encouraged to come forward. It's essential to practice drawing the resistant energy out from deep within the yoni or from the roots of the lingam. When a man notices a high level of arousal in his lover, for instance, instead of *thrusting* to get her to cum, he should do the opposite. He should focus on a passionate outward stroke, rather than the inward thrust. At the same time, he should imagine that he is physically and energetically drawing out her orgasm. The woman, on the other hand, who finds her partner incapable of reaching an orgasm should first gain his trust and cooperation. He must agree to release all goals, as well as fears and thoughts of failure. Then she can take her time and playfully explore every inch of his sexual anatomy, as she searches for his most erogenous zones. Once she discovers his area of vulnerability, she can tease and titillate him, all the while demonstrating her own arousal. Her sexual excitement will often give him permission to release and experience an orgasm.

Some couples find it helpful to create a connection between different parts of the sexual anatomy. To create an association between the yoni and the clitoris or between the prostate and lingam, for example, alternate stimulation between these erogenous zones. To make the association between clitoral or lingam stimulation and orgasm more vivid within the entire body, a man can stroke the inside of the yoni as his partner orgasms through clitoral stimulation. A woman can, on the other hand, stimulate her partner's prostate as he reaches orgasm through stimulation of his lingam. A man can also awaken his partner's yoni by sensually massaging it inside and out, while a woman can bring greater genital awareness to her partner by providing a genital and prostate massage.

Additionally, if a woman is able to reach orgasm through pleasuring but not as easily through intercourse, it is possible to develop an association between the man's lingam and the woman's orgasm by placing his lingam inside her yoni as she is cumming. First stimulate the woman's clitoris to the edge of orgasm, and then slip the lingam into her yoni just prior to orgasm.

Some women find it beneficial to assume a "woman-on-top" position and insert the man's lingam deeply enough to rub his pubic bone against her clitoris. As she rocks her pelvis back and forth, his pubic bone will stimulate her clitoris enough to excite her to orgasm. The clitoral legs (which run along the inside of the inner pelvic bones and along both sides of the vaginal canal) will also feel the rubbing of the lingam, and this added stimulation can trigger a vaginal orgasm simultaneous to the clitoral orgasm.

If a man has more difficulty reaching an orgasm during intercourse than with pleasuring, he too will benefit by his partner's discovering and using the form of stimulation that is most arousing. Then, when he is about to release, they can insert his lingam and bring him to orgasm while thrusting.

If these techniques are practiced consistently, the transmitters of pleasure to the brain connect with the particular part of the body that is stimulated, assisting in a repatterning of pleasure sensations. For example, by connecting the sensations of the clitoris or penis with some other part of the body, that other part soon produces pleasure when stimulated. After developing a pleasure connection between the whole body (or specific parts) and the genitals, it becomes easier for a man or woman to release and surrender to orgasms–especially those of a fuller kind.

TECHNIQUE:
Evoking the Orgasm

One of the best ways to awaken the yoni (especially if the G-spot is dormant) is referred to as "evoking the orgasm."

This technique helps the woman to have push-out contractions, rather than clenching contractions, during her orgasm. Clenching contractions are merely the first level of orgasm for a woman. However, the push-out contractions of an orgasm create a much fuller orgasmic release. Clenching contractions involve only the muscles of the yoni, but push-out contractions involve many pelvic muscles in addition to the vaginal muscles.

During this fuller orgasmic release, the woman feels as though her cervix and uterus are pressing down into the yoni. Usually, these push-out contractions occur only when the woman is in a high state of sexual arousal or after she has experienced some intense orgasms.

STEP 1: While stroking the G-spot inside the vaginal canal, simultaneously stimulate the clitoris with your mouth (or, instead, use two fingers of your other hand).

STEP 2: Continue this dual stimulation until you feel the yoni muscles contracting. When you feel the yoni clenching, simultaneously "pull out" the orgasm with your fingers by *visualizing* it happening and by synchronizing your finger strokes with the contractions of the yoni. Use a beckoning motion and visualize drawing out the orgasm.

STEP 3: Focus your mind on the image or feeling that you are psychically pulling the orgasm out of her yoni.

STEP 4: As the orgasm builds, encourage your partner to occasionally push down gently on her genitals and surrounding muscles, as though she were trying to urinate. This helps to override the tendency to clench the abdominal muscles that results more often in *peak* orgasms and less often in *total-body* orgasms.

Helping Your Partner Orgasm During Intercourse

The lingam has nerve endings throughout its length that become aroused through stimulation. The vaginal wall, on the other hand, has little or no nerve receptors, which explains why most women do not have orgasms exclusively through intercourse. When they do have an orgasm via intercourse, it's usually due to the friction of the lingam against the clitoris or G-spot. However, it is possible to heighten the sensations in a woman's yoni, thus increasing her ability to orgasm through intercourse–even without stimulation to the clitoris.

There are numerous techniques that assist a woman in having an orgasm during intercourse. *First* of all, it's crucial that a woman trusts her partner. *Second*, a woman should relax all of the muscles and tissue within her yoni and body–especially those within the inner vaginal canal. When a woman becomes aroused, she usually tenses the perineum muscle and surrounding pelvic region, causing her vaginal wall to balloon outward. This tensing contracts, or pulls up, the perineum muscle. To reverse the urge to tense or contract, she should push down and out for a moment (with the same muscles she uses for urinating). During intercourse, this act of pushing down collapses the balloon effect, creating a tighter fit of the yoni for the lingam. *Third*, if all else fails, a woman (or her partner) can stimulate her own clitoris manually during intercourse.

Causes Behind the Symptoms

The cells, tissue, and muscles of the body retain, or store, a person's issues. Each person hides different issues in different parts of the body and in various ways. Although no dictionary of emotional ailments could ever assign only one reason for any particular ailment, the list below offers insight into the issues behind some problems in the sexual anatomy.

To add your own ailments and sexual issues to this list, tune into your body and ask what is behind the problem. Try journaling or having a dialog with a specific part of your anatomy to see what your body reveals. Whatever the answers you receive, remember the purpose for this self-investigation is *not* to make you feel worse. It's to help you gain insight into your problem(s), so you can begin a healing process and then surrender it all to God for Divine healing.

FEMALE

ANUS-Subtle attempts to hide insecurities and fears; holding in old hurts.

CLITORIS-Sexual abuse, sexual sadness; waiting for someone to love you deeply enough to open your trust; guilt for faking orgasms; sexual guilt.

VAGINAL CANAL AND UTERUS-Anger at self and others for sexual invasions such as rape, abortions, or childbirth traumas.

BREAST-Resentment for feeling unloved; not embracing your femininity.

MALE

ANUS-Not feeling "good enough" and holding in old hurts.

PENIS–Sexual abuse; issues with self-worth and masculinity.

PROSTATE–Guilt about overusing one's sexuality or insecurity about using it at all.

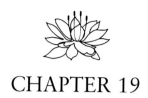

CHAPTER 19

Sacred Sexual Gatherings

The Sacred Puja

Group sex may be the most controversial part of any book on sexuality, as it involves sexual activities that can easily be misconstrued as orgies. This section of the book, however, is not promoting such activities. It is merely presenting sexual gatherings as options that can be conducted with love and integrity.

The topic of sexual gatherings is a vital part of the history of sacred sexuality. Ancient cultures have demonstrated that, if done with an elevated intent, such gatherings can be spiritually powerful and result in the experience and integration of ecstatic, loving energy. **The difference between a sacred sexual gathering and an orgy is the focus of intent–the same criterion for discerning *lovemaking* from *having sex* and *self-loving* from merely *masturbating*.**

A sacred sexual gathering can take many different forms. But whether three or thirty people share in a gathering, the theme and intent must always be clear, understood, and upheld. Indeed, one of the primary purposes behind such gatherings is the development of the self-discipline necessary for the participants to hold their focus despite the obvious potential distractions. Again, the form and details of how such a gathering materializes can vary based on the individuals and their philosophical beliefs. Yet such themes as love, healing, responsibility, trust, and acceptance must remain present for the gathering to be truly a sacred space.

One common ego-oriented pitfall that can surface during sacred sexual gatherings involves the judging of other people–on any level, including physical appearance. Therefore, to preserve the sacredness of the gathering, everyone's thoughts and words should convey love and respect for all others.

Jealousy, another common obstacle to the success of loving relationships, is also a potential pitfall at sacred sexual gatherings.

Jealousy is perhaps the most debilitating...of emotions. Jealousy is concerned with possessing and controlling another person; it is not an expression of love.

–Diana Richardson *(Tantric Orgasm for Women)*

The sanctity of privacy is another concern at a sacred sexual gathering. **There is a difference between** *privacy* **and** *secrecy*, **the latter usually involves lying and sneaking, while the former involves respecting boundaries.** Respecting the privacy of others requires and encourages all participants to develop trust. Everything shared in a sacred sexual gathering must be honored as private, unless otherwise agreed upon by all persons concerned.

In Tantra, a group ceremony is referred to as a *"puja."* When done correctly, a *puja* incorporates the highest spiritual ideals into an intimate group setting. Its purpose is to transcend the boundaries of social norm, dissolve possessiveness, eliminate jealousy, and put the greater good of the group before any personal agendas. When these ideals are achieved, the rewards are profound and healing for all of the participants who willingly drop their egos and surrender to the power of joining in oneness.

TECHNIQUE:

A Sacred Sexual Gathering (Puja)

The attendees of a true sacred sexual gathering are (and must remain) spiritually mature and emotionally responsible. Their thoughts and intentions are necessarily focused on sharing love and experiencing bliss. Attitudes or emotions that are incongruent with this focus could undermine the atmosphere and spiritual presence desired by the group and necessary to achieve the purpose of the gathering. Participants must therefore remain aware of their inner processings. Any personal issues should be handled appropriately and not be permitted to "spill over" into the sacred circle, acting as an energetic virus to the other participants.

The most excellent place for practicing men is wherever there is a gathering of practicing women; there, all the magical powers will be attained.

—*Cakrasamvara Tantra*

Whether a group is small or large, in order to maintain the highest intent (holding a focus of love, while avoiding the most common distractions of inhibitions and jealous competition), love must be equal between all parties involved.

The following is one example of the steps for creating a sacred sexuality gathering, or puja:

STEP 1: Make the floor comfortable with lots of padding (blankets, pillows, and/or mattresses).

STEP 2: Prepare the environment with aroma, music, water, massage oils, snacks, and condoms (if agreed upon). Sanctify and purify the room. Burn a few candles, preferably aromatic.

STEP 3: Have all participants thoroughly cleanse their entire bodies or, better yet, bathe, dry, and then anoint each other with oil. Next, adorn each other with flowers, scarves, and jewelry, as if giving an offering to royalty or a deity.

STEP 4: Open with a prayer of dedication. Ask to feel the Divine Presence throughout your being and to awaken as a god or goddess. Then bring your centered presence to the group. Throughout the remainder of the ceremony, women take on the embodiment of Shakti, while men become Shiva.

STEP 5: Offer your partner(s) gifts of drink and a snack of fruit or another form of refreshing, sensual food.

STEP 6: Share a group sacred dance (slow, fast, or a combination of both) or perhaps a few yoga asanas. Culminate this dance with all participants rubbing and charging each other with ecstatic energy.

STEP 7: When the dancing is complete, sit or stand with a partner, hold hands or embrace with your arms, make eye contact, verbally acknowledge something you love and/or appreciate about that person and then hum together. The humming might evolve into toning or chanting, but don't force it.

STEP 8: Invite at least one other person to the floor and sensually massage each other. Begin lightly (in order to create a connection), and then massage deeper to release any tensions in the muscles that could inhibit energy flow. Switch partners until everyone has given and received.

STEP 9: Now give and receive sensual touch and stimulation using your hair, fingertips, and other tools to awaken your partner's body, especially the breasts and genitals. As you receive, be sure to give voice to natural moans and sighs. Playfully kiss, lick, suck, and rub, but do not bring your partner to orgasm. Merely use this playfulness to build more sexual energy.

STEP 10: Enjoy watching and hearing the arousal of others. Take the arousal into your body, and allow the beauty of others to ignite a greater awakening of energy within *you*. Eventually give yourself permission to let go and "get physical." Be accepting of your desires as well as those of others.

STEP 11: Let yourself feel wild and uninhibited. Build toward orgasm but choose not to "go over the edge." Once orgasmic energy builds sufficiently, you can rearrange the bodies of you and your partner into the yab yum position (the woman sitting on her partner's lap) and practice in-jaculation and energy circulation exercises.

STEP 12: You might choose to insert the lingam into the yoni, but this is optional. If the lingam *is* inserted, occasionally move your pelvises to further increase arousal. Gently rock your bodies back and forth. Shiva (the man) exhales, as he sends energy from his lingam into Shakti's (the woman's) yoni and up to her crown chakra. Simultaneously, Shakti inhales and imagines drawing her partner's sexual energy into her yoni and up to her crown chakra.

STEP 13: Then this process is reversed. As Shakti exhales, she sends energy from her crown to her genitals and up into Shiva's crown chakra. Shiva simultaneously inhales and draws this energy into his genitals and up to his crown. One is inhaling and drawing energy in, while the other is exhaling and sending energy out. In other words, there is a flow of energy from your crown to your genitals and then from your genitals to your partner's crown. Then back from your partner's crown and genitals and into your genitals and crown again. This cycle can be repeated for several minutes.

STEP 14: Build as much orgasmic energy as possible. When you feel energy circulate up your spine, filling your meridians and nervous system, occasionally shake your body and limbs to prevent energy blocks. Playfully pretend that you are feeling orgasms and moan freely as you do. This imaginative playfulness, in itself, is freeing and healing of inhibitions. Then laugh, smile, and shake your body and limbs again.

STEP 15: If the feeling arises and you choose to have a physical release (orgasm), do so at any time. Or have more than one.

STEP 16: After you have built sufficient ecstatic energy (and perhaps have had an orgasm), lie still, relaxed, tension free, and as comfortable as possible. Then allow the ecstatic energy to move through you, which may feel like waves or occasional jolts of electricity. Take your time and enjoy the afterglow as a deep state of quiet meditation. Remain quiet and still as you feel a spirit of oneness with your partner(s) and the group as a whole.

STEP 17: Close with a prayer of thanks. Share lots of hugs of gratitude.

STEP 18: Do some grounding stretches to integrate the energy and experience into your body. Then take time to wash each other.

IMPORTANT REMINDERS
FOR SACRED GATHERINGS (PUJAS)

When sharing such vulnerable aspects of your being with others, especially as a group, some *very* clear rules and guidelines are necessary. Begin by reviewing the goals and essentials of sacred sexuality, as noted in the introduction of this book. Other guidelines are as follows:

- Remain in your spiritual center and intention as much as possible. Remind *yourself* to allow the Divine Presence of God to experience through you.

- Enjoy all sensations, large and small. Moan in appreciation of these sensations.

- Release all thoughts of judgements, goals, and agendas.

- If fears or personal issues arise, move yourself to the side of the room, and do some praying and releasing. Then, if or when you feel the time is right, begin self-stimulating and/or move back into the group.

Sensual Manifestation Ceremony

Everything within the universe is filled with pure, creative energy. Through our minds' use of focused love, we access this energy and alter the form of the universe (and of our lives), thus becoming participants in a co-creation process. Sexual energy is one of the most powerful tools, or vehicles, for focusing and projecting our creative, loving thoughts. Orgasmic energy combined with heightened awareness can be harnessed to magnify these creative inspirations. In order to master this co-creative process, individuals must learn to properly utilize their sexual arousal and threshold of orgasm.

TECHNIQUE:
Seven-Step Manifestation Ritual

When individuals join with others who have a similar intent of synchronizing creative love-power and collective orgasm, they can build up an intense level of energetic ecstasy that can be channeled into creative manifestation.

Whether for an individual or a group, sexual creative power is magnified by activating the body's senses; therefore, it is wise to stimulate as many of the senses as possible in a sexual ceremony designed for a group. Use flavors in the mouth for *taste*, aromas for *scent*, music and moans for *sound*, massage and caressing for *touch*, and most of all, *visual* scenes for creating greater arousal. In addition to increasing arousal, activating the senses helps individuals remain focused and present.

Once again, a group sexual gathering (or ceremony) might be judged by some as a mere orgy with shallow intentions. As with anything in life, sexual ceremonies can be misused, but when shared properly, these rituals have proven very powerful for ancient and modern practitioners.

STEP 1: OPENING PRAYERS–Prayerfully affirm God's loving Presence. State your intent (what you wish to manifest in your life), and then keep this intention in the back of your mind throughout the manifestation ritual.

STEP 2: ACTIVATING AROUSAL–Stimulate your genitals and erogenous zones. After you are slightly aroused, begin stimulating the bodies of other participants in the ceremony. Use rhythm, dance, touch, moans and perhaps even sexual penetration to build sexual arousal.

STEP 3: INTENSIFICATION–Build up the ecstasy towards orgasm, but do not go over the edge into full release. Practice self-control. Re-focus on your intent for manifestation.

STEP 4: INITIAL ORGASM–Become vividly familiar with the time and space between knowing the orgasm has arrived and the point of the first release. For most people this is a fraction of a second, but it needs to be paused and expanded. Once again, draw your attention to your initial focus and intent. Relax and bask in the excitation. Repeat the cycle of building arousal and postponing ejaculation.

STEP 5: ORGASM–This is the second part of the orgasm. Use your willpower to slow down all forms of stimulation, prolong the orgasmic release, and expand your focus beyond bodily sensations. You may experience an ejaculation, or you may experience orgasms of ecstasy without actually ejaculating. Either way, during all forms of ecstatic release, deepen your breath and visualize the results of your intended manifestation. Use the power of the orgasm to further *intensify* the image of your intent. Use all of this heightened arousal, energy, and focus to imagine the fruition of your prayer. The more intense the orgasm, the more you must use your willpower to maintain the image of your visualization.

STEP 6: RIDING THE WAVE–After the orgasm begins to dissipate, connect your breathing with feelings of calmness. Simultaneously hold feelings of appreciation, knowing that the object of your imaging has now become a blueprint from which the universe will create the manifestation of your intent. Maintain occasional, but gentle, physical stimulation while keeping your mind focused. You have stated your prayer; now let God send images, symbols, and messages to you. Allow a visual journey to unfold.

STEP 7: COMING DOWN–Soak up the experience. Slow your breathing and stretch your body. Engage in light conversation, humming or moaning, as well as light massage and grounding exercises. Once again, re-focus on your intent and give thanks.

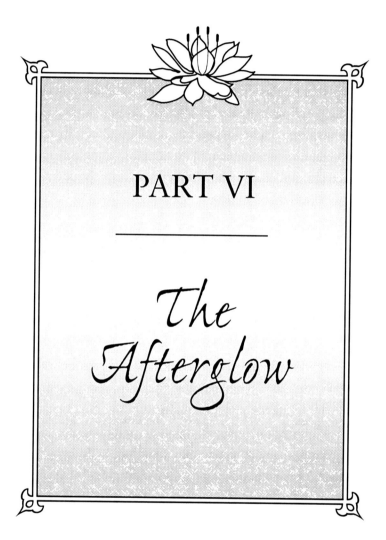

PART VI

The Afterglow

Postplay

The afterglow is as much an essential part of the sacred sexual experience as any step leading up to this moment. The *postplay*, or afterglow, can be viewed as the opposite of *foreplay* because it involves "coming down," as opposed to "building up." Yet the afterglow has many of the same ingredients as foreplay *and* the actual sexual encounter–such as being present, communicating, connecting, and even physical contact. If properly treated, the afterglow can prolong the mood created during the precious moments of any sexual experience.

Sacred sexuality doesn't end with an orgasm or with the ecstatic experience of feeling waves of energy and universal love. Instead, the sacred sexual experience (like all sacred experiences) is meant to be integrated into your life and being–becoming a part of who and what you are. The time of postplay is a perfect opportunity to experience this integration.

During the afterglow, both partners are experiencing absorption of fluidic essences and a continuing exchange of energy. After the energy subsides, it's then time to share thoughts, feelings, and experiences. Later, the feeling of intimacy can be prolonged while washing up–perhaps with a sensual shower together. Even when it's time to get dressed, you can playfully assist each other, which continues the feeling of love, respect, and sacredness.

As communication helps to integrate all that was gained from the sexual experience into your relationship, grounding exercises help to integrate the energy from the sexual experience into the cells of your body. Therefore, getting grounded (and into your body) before attempting to interact with the outside world is the final stage of postplay and afterglow. All of the elements of foreplay (communicating, connecting, and grounding) make for an integrated experience that has permanent effects on your mind, body, and soul.

As can be seen, the repertoire for postplay involves more than just holding each other. Postplay also includes coming down, remaining present, connecting, expressing appreciation, cleaning up, communicating, and integrating.

The last chapter (Chapter 20) in this book offers applicable ideas and techniques for creating a more fulfilling "afterglow." In some regards, the afterglow is the most commonly missed part of lovemaking, and again, is easily as important as any other.

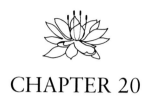

CHAPTER 20

Closure

Coming Down

During the "coming down" phase of the sexual experience, lovers slowly regain their composure, and their breathing gradually returns to normal. Usually they experience a heightened state of relaxation and an inner state of calmness.

In some respects, the coming down phase is experienced alone, yet in other respects, it's experienced with your partner. Each partner needs to have "space" to release any leftover tension and absorb the continuing waves of energy. Then, gradually, as the lovers focus back into their present surroundings, they will be capable of being more present with each other.

"Ecstasy is characterized by extreme peace, tranquility, serenity and radiant joy. [It is] a blissful, tension-free state, a loss of ego boundaries and an absolute sense of oneness with nature, with the cosmic order, and with God."

–Stanislav Grof

Remaining Present

The concept of "being present" has been mentioned throughout this book as vital to any sacred sexual experience. But it's equally essential at the *closing* of a sexual encounter. By not rushing off into life's distraction–by remaining focused and present–now more than ever, you can demonstrate to your partner that he or she is a priority to you. This may be one of the most important messages you ever offer your partner.

Holding and Connecting

Be sure to hold each other and snuggle after a sacred sexual experience. Perhaps you can tend to each other's needs by serving water or feeding each other cool, fresh fruit. Or assist with some preliminary washing of each other's bodies.

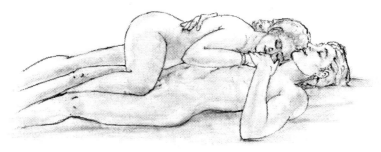

Holding and connecting

Generally, this vital moment of connecting is stereotypically considered to be more important to a woman than a man. Women are said to more often request being held after intercourse and miss it when it's not provided. If this is true, then the way a man deals with the afterglow period reveals much about his personal nature and psychological health. For example, if he falls asleep or rushes from the room, it might indicate a fear of deeper connecting, as well as unhealed phobias or negative beliefs about sex. Of course, just because he hangs around a little longer doesn't mean he's a saint–especially if he is doing so just to get more sex. But his ability to maintain a conscious presence after sex can reveal his commitment to a deeper, more authentic connection with his partner.

Again, for some women, holding and connecting can be virtually the most important part of any sexual experience. In fact, women often participate in sex simply to achieve a deeper level of connection and, sometimes, just for the holding–a need many men rarely fulfill.

Expressing Gratitude

Now is your chance to assure your partner that all the effort he or she put into co-creating the sacred sexual experience was well worth it and appreciated. Do everything in your power to articulate and demonstrate how wonderful the experience was and how much you appreciate the sharing. Your appreciation can be conveyed through thoughts, words, and/or gestures.

Cleaning Up

Cleaning up after a sexual encounter is a delicate matter. You don't want to send your partner signals that imply you are ashamed of, or turned-off by, the remnants of lovemaking. However, it is wise for health reasons to cleanse the genitals as soon as possible after sex–particularly if oral sex is involved. This cleansing helps to reduce the chance of germ-related viruses and irritations. Since some women have an allergy to latex, be sure to wash off any residue if a condom was used.

Communicating

It's best not to rush into talking immediately after intimate encounters. Nevertheless, communication is helpful for both partners. Communication should always be loving, tactful, and accentuate the positives. It might be best to focus primarily on what worked well. Wait until later to discuss what you wanted more of, or what could be improved, to avoid the impression of complaining. Absorb all feedback and allow it to enhance your knowledge and understanding of your partner (and yourself).

Integrating and Grounding

The integration process encompasses absorbing the love, energy, and essence of the experience shared with your partner. In some respects, integration is accomplished through the aforementioned stages of the postplay process–coming down, being present, connecting, gratitude, and communication. However, the integration process also includes cleaning up together, dressing each other, and doing grounding exercises.

Becoming grounded helps you feel centered and present. It prevents the sleepiness some people experience after sex. It also prevents spaciness and integrates the aroused sexual energy into the bloodstream. The most basic form of grounding exercises involves slow yoga-like stretches–particularly of the legs. When doing grounding stretches or breathing, envision your legs as roots that ground you (the tree) to the earth.

EXERCISE:

Grounding Stretch

Of all the grounding exercises commonly practiced, this one, although possibly the easiest, is by far the most effective. As with all grounding exercises, the primary purpose is to channel the body's energy downward toward the feet. In so doing, it alleviates spaciness, while creating a sense of being in the "here and now."

1. Stand with your feet at shoulders' width apart.
2. Bend forward at the waist (bringing your hands as close to the ground as possible). Place your palms on the ground and straighten your legs. If you cannot straighten them, it's fine to have them slightly bent.
3. Slowly stretch the back of your legs for two or three minutes.
4. When you are done stretching, you should notice a slight trembling in the legs and yet a sense of feeling grounded and present in the moment.

EXERCISE:

Grounding Breath

While the previous exercise might be an effective *stretch* for grounding, the following is the most common *breathing* exercise for grounding. This exercise utilizes the "hara," the chakra commonly known as the naval center and the body's center of gravity. In martial arts, the hara is termed the center of gravity because whenever a practitioner's attention moves above the naval center, he (or she) is easily tripped or thrown.

1. Sit comfortably or stand with your feet at shoulders' width and knees slightly bent.
2. Begin inhaling slow, deep breaths as you draw energy from the ethers

around you and down into your hara (naval center—two inches below your naval).

3. On the exhale, visualize sending the energy of your breath down into your legs and continuing into the earth.

4. Repeat this grounding exercise at least three times.

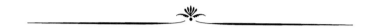

The sensual pleasure women provide, the joy of wine, the taste of meat: it is the undoing of fools, but for the wise, the pathway to salvation.

–Kalarnava Tantra

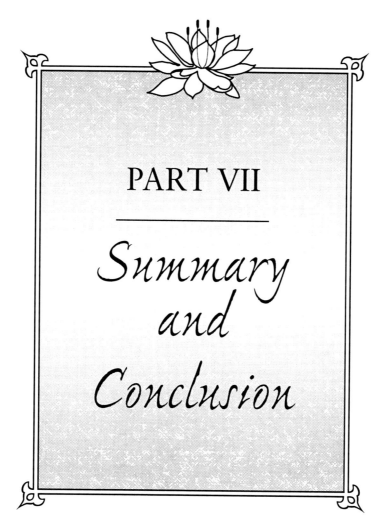

PART VII

Summary
and
Conclusion

Now for the Best Part

Imagine for a moment how your life (and sexual experiences) might have been different if you had been taught the concepts of sacred sexuality when you were a teenager. Chances are you will agree that your life would have been *very* different.

If you have read and absorbed any part of this book, you have already begun to integrate its information and goals. The more you integrate and practice the concepts taught, the more your life will change. You will have moments where you feel ecstatically alive and in harmony with your sexuality—a vital key to your health and well-being. Reading the conclusion of this book can coincide with a new beginning for you. So allow the application and integration of this material to take you from *knowledge* in your mind to *awareness* in your soul. You will then emerge more spiritually connected and physically alive.

What is really so heartbreaking is that God has been with me all along, And I simply avoided His Presence. Yet now I can feel Him inside my heart, as closely as I feel my partner.

–Valerie Brooks *(Tantric Awakening)*

As you learn to balance and integrate the spiritual and physical aspects of your being, you will reach a level of empowerment of which most people only dream. You may find that others are attracted to you on various levels, so remember to maintain your center. Instead of responding to every attraction to or from others, empower *them* by being true to *yourself.* Demonstrate how to be loving, sensual, and passionate, yet responsible. Show others **it is possible to be fully alive in your body without compromising your soul.** Let others know that you see the wonderful qualities in them, as well as in yourself. You can choose to occasionally share your love and passion with others, but be clear that they must earn the right to touch your body (as you must earn the right to touch theirs). The body is the temple of the soul. It is sacred. *You* are sacred!

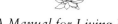

Throughout this book there have been reminders that, although the content speaks of sexuality, its goal is not sex, in and of itself. **Ultimately, this book uses sex as a metaphor for spiritual connection or, at the least, as an arena for such a connection.** The intent is not to get you more caught-up in your body, your senses or shallow pleasures. In truth, you are *not* and do not *have* a body. If you really did, your body would rule and limit you, but it does not, even though most of us believe to the contrary. Since you are not a body, sacred sexuality urges you to expand your awareness, connection, and understanding of who and what you are. Through use of the body, you are urged to discover a love and peace that surpasses the body's comprehension.

We are glorious, spiritual beings capable of experiencing bliss beyond the body's ability to contain. Therefore, all the thoughts, words, exercises, and techniques in this book, which seem to focus on the body and its sensations, are but the momentary honoring of the physical illusion. In other words, this book merely uses the body and sexuality as means for remembering the truth of the spirit. The sacred sexual experience becomes an arena in which to be playful, spontaneous, nonjudgmental, and above all, loving. This happens to be a perfect description for living a Divine embodiment. Sacred sexuality therefore returns us to the Garden of Eden, where we unite our hearts and souls with other people who are on the same journey Home. The sacred sexual experience is really about a remembrance that **we are the embodiment of the Love behind, and beyond, lovemaking.**

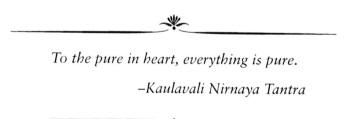

To the pure in heart, everything is pure.

–*Kaulavali Nirnaya Tantra*

PART VIII

Appendix

An Outline of a Sacred Sexual Experience

The following chart provides a basic outline of a sacred sexual encounter. It can be photocopied and memorized or kept near at hand as a lovemaking guide.

I. SELF AWARENESS

1. Personal Centering and Self Observation–Loosen up the body and get centered.
2. Personal Hygiene–Cleanse your body thoroughly.
3. Self-Awareness–Acknowledge and prayerfully surrender any arising issues and inhibitions.
4. Visualization–Envision the kind of intimate encounter you would like to experience.

II. INTIMACY WITH OTHERS

1. Preparation–Prepare the environment. Include some candles, water, and perhaps fresh fruit.
2. Dedication–Take a moment to share some prayer or call in Divine Presence and acknowledge the divinity in yourself and your partner.
3. Cleansing–Take time to wash your body and sanitize your mouth.
4. Communication and Connecting–Discuss intent, boundaries, and preferences.
5. Massaging and Caressing–Practice variations of initial contact, massage, and genital stimulation.
6. Kissing and Mouthplay–Indulge in kissing, licking, and biting.
7. Oral Sex–Pleasure your partner as a buildup for intercourse *or* to the point of orgasm itself.

III. INTERCOURSE

1. Variations of Positions–Find the positions that work best for you and your lover.
2. Ejaculation Control–Practice the building up and holding off of orgasm.

3. Self-Awareness–Use various techniques to evoke orgasms.

4. Expand the Energy of the Orgasm–Whether you choose ejaculation or not, slow the orgasmic energy to spread it throughout your body.

IV. AFTERGLOW

1. Coming Down–Remain present and gracious.

2. Connecting–Take time to hold each other and connect.

3. Cleanup–Wash up or shower together.

4. Post-sex Communication–Discuss the experience and share feedback.

5. Grounding–Do stretches or take a walk to get grounded.

Terminology

The following is a clarification of terms used in this book. Some of the words listed are ancient Sanskrit, while others are Taoist. Each of these words includes a translation. In addition to the terms derived from ancient languages, this list also includes commonly used "crude" sexual slang along with the origins of such words. The purpose of including crude slang in a list of sacred terms is to enlighten the reader as to how seemingly *irrational* "street terms" often have *rational* origins.

Asanas–A Sanskrit term for yoga postures *or* sexual positions. Symbolic body mudras, that place the practitioner in a receptive mode to receive Spirit.

Bandhas–(or locks) Specific muscle contraction exercises designed to seal off particular segments of the body, thus channeling energy into the desired segments of the body.

Blow Job–"Blo" is an old English term for prostitute. (slang for "fellatio," or the oral pleasuring performed on a man's genitals).

Chakras–Sanskrit word for spinning wheel, or energy vortex, within the body that draws life-force from the ethers and into the body's organs and meridians.

Clitoris–(or jewel) A penis-like appendage that sits outside and above the opening of the vagina. It comes from the root word *clavis*, which means "key." The clitoris is clearly a key to a woman's experience of sexual pleasure and release.

Cock–Slang terminology for the erect, male penis, or lingam. It means "lifted and prepared to fire."

Cum (not "come")–From "a-*cum*-mulated" energy or substance. It refers to the energetic and fluidic release during orgasm.

Cunnilingus–The oral pleasuring performed on a woman's genitals.

Cunt–From *cunni,* which is a reference to the vagina. *Cunni* means "vagina."

Dakini–A Tantric guardian of the deeper mysteries. It usually refers to the female partner in the Tantric initiations or any human female who has achieved high levels of wisdom and awareness and is thereafter referred to as a goddess or *dakini.* The closest English version of the term would be "living angel" or "lightworker." All goddesses can be referred to as *dakini*, which means "sky walking woman." The male equivalent is referred to as a *daka*.

Deva–Sanskrit word for "god." *Devi* is a Sanskrit word for "goddess."

Ejaculation–Male ejaculations include the emission of semen, sperm, pre-cum, and other fluids upon orgasm. Female ejaculations are not experienced by all women; but when they occur, the ejaculate is made up of prostatic fluids from the paraurethral glands, fluids from the Bartholin glands, urine, fluids from the fallopian tubes, and other miscellaneous fluids.

Fellatio–The oral pleasuring performed on a man's genitals.

FUCK–Fornication Under Consent of King. (slang for "intercourse")

G-spot–Originally called the "Grafenberg Spot"–also commonly referred to as the "G-oddess Spot." The G-spot is the female equivalent of the prostate and greatly contributes to vaginal (non-clitoral) orgasms, which occasionally include ejaculations in some women. Female ejaculations release fluids primarily from the paraurethral glands and ducts, located alongside of the female urethra, a region known as the urethral sponge.

In-jaculation–Turning an ejaculation inward.

Lingam–Sanskrit for "Wand of Light," referring to an erect penis. Another Tantric term for the penis is *vajra*, which means "thunderbolt." In Taoism–"Jade Stem" or "Jade Stalk."

Maithuna–A traditional, ritual practice of lovemaking.

Mantra–Sanskrit meaning "to focus the mind." A mantra is a sacred syllable or phrase that is repeated to focus the mind on the object of desire or worship.

Nadis–Term used in Tantra and yoga to indicate invisible "veins" that channel energy throughout the body to all organs and chakras. In Tantric tradition, it is believed that the body has 14 major nadis and 72,000 general nadis. The most important three (of the 14 major) nadis–running along the spine from tailbone to head–are sushumna, the central channel; ida, the left, feminine channel that ends in the left nostril; and pingala, the right, masculine channel that ends in the right nostril.

Namaste–A Hindu greeting that loosely translates as, "I honor God within you and within me."

Om Mani Padme Hum–*Om* calls on the higher realms, *Mani* acknowledges the male principle, *Padme* acknowledges the female principle, and *Hum* refers to turning within oneself. It also translates as, "Like a jewel in the center of the lotus, God is in the heart of me."

Orgasm–Means "to swell with excitement." It derives from the same root word as "orgy."

Panchamakara–Commonly known as the Tantric ritual of "the Five M's." This ritual involves several (usually at least eight) men and women practicing five traditional observances or rituals of partaking. In left-hand Tantra, they use *madya* (wine), *mamsa* (meat), *matsya* (fish), *mudra* and *maithuna*. In some schools of right-hand Tantra, they substitute with coconut juice, cheese, ginger, rice and honey.

Penis–A clinical term for the male organ/shaft.

Puja–Sanskrit for a sacred gathering or ceremony. In some styles of tantra, a *puja* involves a group gathering, rituals, prayers, and worship but can also include sexual interaction.

Pussy–Cat fur–once used for masturbation (slang for "vagina").

Sanskrit–An ancient root language used throughout India and other parts of Asia and therefore the primary language used in ancient Hindu Tantra and modern Western Tantra.

Shakti–A goddess and Shiva's consort in the Tantric tradition. Also female sexual energy.

Shiva–A god in the Tantric tradition. He is said to take on three forms–one of which is the lingam.

Tantra–Sanskrit for an art or tool for joining or weaving together.

Tantric Texts–Tantric scriptures are generally classified as either Hindu or Buddhist "Tantras." Although many of the original *Tantras* have been lost, there are several that still exist as translations. Besides the original *Tantras*, there are also several well-known classic texts that describe the practice of Tantra and sacred sexuality. Not nearly as old as the original *Tantras*, they include (1) the *Kama Sutra*, written by Vatsyayana, an ancient Indian text that served as a sex manual and has become the most famous of all Indian erotic works; (2) the *Ananga Ranga*, written by Kalyanamalla, which, similar to the *Kama Sutra*, deals with a variety of erotic and sexual subjects ranging from aphrodisiacs to sexual positions and the art of seduction; and (3) *The Perfumed Garden*, an Arabian work written by Sheikh Nefzaoui. *The Perfumed Garden* includes several erotic tales, as well as describing numerous sexual positions and techniques.

Yantra– A Sanskrit term for a sacred geometric symbol (similar to a mandala), infused with energy and used to enhance a practitioner's concentration, thus magnifying the effects of his or her Tantric practices.

Yoni–Sanskrit for "Sacred Space"–the female sexual organs or vagina. In Taoism–"Jade Cavern" or "Jade Gate."

Sexual Facts

This list is compiled from the latest research and surveys. While such facts are never a hundred percent accurate, the statements are nevertheless generally true. These details are certain to evoke varied responses and interpretations. It is possible to perceive a pattern of evolution regarding sexuality, demonstrated by the fact that in the last twenty years twice as many women report having orgasms. This is a quantum leap towards freedom from the sexual "dark ages." On the other hand, it might appear that we still have a need for greater sexual healing and education, which is demonstrated by the fact that ninety percent of teenagers in most high schools claim to have already had sex. Furthermore, most of the teenagers surveyed have reported that they failed to use condoms.

Aside from pointing out some dramatic facts about sex and sexuality, this information can also dispel misconceptions on the topic. It may prove comforting to know where you stand in relation to the statistics. It may also serve to motivate you to make some changes in your sexual experiences. If you find any of the noted facts to be doubtful, simply check the Internet or your local library resource center.

1. Over 90% of men and 70% of women masturbate.
2. Although women *are* capable of sexual pleasure, orgasm, and even ejaculation, this fact is still doubted by medical science.
3. Only 14% of women report having multiple orgasms.
4. As much as 37% of males have had at least one homosexual experience.
5. Only one out of ten women report a wonderful first sexual experience.
6. Only 30% of women report reaching orgasm during sexual intercourse, but over 80% reach orgasm during masturbation.
7. Sexually active adults worldwide have sex on an average of once every three days.
8. Nearly 50% of the world's adults have had a one-night stand.
9. Nearly 60% of women surveyed have faked an orgasm and just 15% of men.
10. As many as one-in-ten sexually active adults have had sex with their best friend's partner.
11. The average male reaches orgasm within five minutes.

12. The average male orgasm lasts only three seconds.

13. The average male penis is 3 inches (when not erect) and 5-6 inches (when erect).

14. The average depth of a woman's vagina is only about 4 inches, but it elongates during intercourse.

15. Well over half of all men and women surveyed report having experimented with such minor forms of bondage as wrist binding and blindfolding.

16. Well over half of all men and women surveyed report having experimented with some form of sex toy.

17. Less than 30% of sexually active adults report feeling comfortable talking dirty.

18. Although 75% of men have orgasms with their partners, only 30% of women can make the same claim.

19. By the age of fifty, nearly 40% of all males and 20% of females will have had an affair.

20. One in every three sexually active people will contract an STD by the age of thirty-five.

21. Recent reports claim that over 90% of high school students in the USA have had intercourse.

22. Nearly one-in-four women have been forced to perform a sexual act

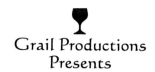

Grail Productions
Presents

Exploring Sacred Sexuality

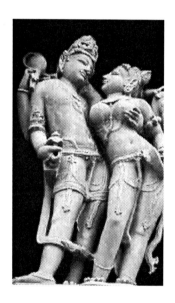

Facilitated by Michael Mirdad, this workshop is a five-day intensive that synthesizes the most effective arts of sacred sexuality, including Tantra and Taoist sexology. This workshop also incorporates modern techniques of sexual healing. The event is for everyone: whether you are single, have a partner, are sexually active or not. In the safest and most sacred atmosphere, you will learn to develop and channel your own sexual energy to enhance health, vitality and self awareness.

THE WORKSHOP ALSO FEATURES:

- An introduction to sexual anatomy and terminology

- Tantric and Taoist techniques to enhance your sexual experience

- Techniques for channeling your sexual energy into creative ecstasy

- Exercises for health, vitality, and rejuvenation

- Techniques for enhancing the intimacy in your relationships

- Self-awareness to heal sexual guilt, shame, and inhibitions

To apply for this workshop, please contact us at:

Grail Productions, PO Box 2783, Bellingham, WA 98227
For information: 360-671-8349 or grailpro@aol.com.
Visit us at **www.SacredSexuality.US**

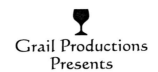

Grail Productions
Presents

— WORKSHOP FEEDBACK —

Of all the workshops I've ever attended or participated in, this is by far the most life altering I have ever experienced. It demonstrated the incredible connection to Spirit we all have within us. I was overwhelmed with the depth and authenticity of the other attendees and consider it such a gift from above. Words like authentic, spiritual, delicious, integrity, sensual, playful, amazing, sacred, and powerful all seem to be not enough to bring forth the essence of this workshop. I enjoyed working with and discovering the tumescence energy of the body. I have been fascinated by energy work and studying it for years and in one short demonstration it all came together for me! Since the workshop, I feel a constant humming sound of contentment as well as heightened senses. –**Dawn, AK**

The Sacred Sexuality workshop was the best investment, and gift, that I have ever given to myself. I am still on cloud 9 (the Afterglow), and I am doing my best not to let it end. As I am writing this, and thinking about the loving energy of all who attended, tears of joy are filling my eyes. Just saying thank you cannot begin to express how grateful I am to God for bringing such a wonderful group of people together, and to you Michael for allowing God to work through you, to help us reconnect with ourselves and others through unconditional love. The weekend workshop was an eye opening experience for me in many ways. I learned that in letting go of judgments and fears we can reach a state of intoxicating euphoria that I never knew existed. I also learned that allowing myself to receive unconditional love is just as wonderful as giving. Other people are seeing the glow as well and they're smiling in response. –**Carmen, FL**

At the Sacred Sexuality workshop I discovered freedom and self-love and learned to experience my body in a safe and loving manner. I enjoyed bonding with women and experiencing a sense of sisterhood. I feel so alive and beautiful. –**Traci, AK**

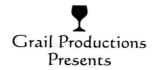

Grail Productions
Presents

— WORKSHOP FEEDBACK —

I experienced healing in all areas of my life, emotionally, spiritually and sexually. I have a clearer understanding of how my fears hold me back from participating in so many things life has to offer. I could never have envisioned all that I experienced and felt at the Sacred Sexuality intensive. The pace and layout of the workshop could not have been better. Michael certainly has a gift of knowing what to do, when and how. He demonstrated how to be fully present, in tune and thoughtful throughout the event. –Beverly, TX

Last night as I was drifting off to sleep and reminiscing about the Sacred Sexuality workshop, I remembered holding, being held, love touching me beyond words, and dancing with all of my new friends. I can still feel the frolicking energy, playful beings, souls with purpose...God in skin. Dancing so many dances, light bouncing playful; stomping; writhing; teasing; losing self; floating in the space; laughter, smiles, and joy. I also remember looking into the depths of each soul. I am excited about learning more and putting it into practice. The love I experienced at the workshop has helped me to know who I will choose to share my body with. I guess it hit home how precious or delicate I really am. I also learned to go beyond our bodies, seeing past all the skin. Focusing on the packaging of people is simply a way to keep distance from the light within each of us. So, by watching others, looking into everyone's eyes, feeling their breath, seeing everyone as 'spirit' helped me realize I am not my packaging either. And treating myself any other way only limits my connection with others. – Tanya, AK

This workshop is amazing. Every man on the planet should attend. The incredible healings that occurred for me still continue to astound me. There was a point in the workshop where I thought, "This must have been what it was like in the Garden of Eden" and I felt like a child playing in that garden. –Ron, CANADA

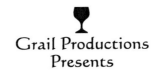

Grail Productions
Presents

— WORKSHOP FEEDBACK —

I don't know where to start! I am now capable of being comfortable around a man. I also learned that my own body and sexual anatomy are beautiful. My trust and safety have grown to a great extent. I feel so incredibly happy and sometimes feel like a little girl–so happy to be alive and very, very happy with who I am. I find myself jumping around, dancing naked, and loving my body. Other times I feel much more mature and understanding myself at a deeper level. I feel grounded and free. Even my relationships with others are great, as if they understand where I am right now. It's as if by accepting myself, other people are doing so as well. It feels like in this workshop I worked in so many areas of myself–physical, emotional, mental, and spiritual. I feel free to "feel" my body. I feel like exploring it and I really like what I have been finding! –J B, Mexico

Attending the Sacred Sexuality workshop taught me to accept my feelings about sexuality without judgment and to understand myself and others with more love, compassion, and sensitivity. I learned to integrate God with my sexuality. The workshop challenged my old opinions and beliefs and showed me how much they influenced my life. But I am now more open and clear about what I want within my own boundaries and am open to learn and stretch. I feel clearer about my sexuality and that my heart, and mind are all positively affected together, as this life-force flows through me. I feel powerful knowing that I get to choose how I express and experience my sexuality–which is now sacred. –Jackie, ONT

It was such a blessing to join in playfulness and reverence for God with the shared intent of remembering who we really are. In addition, there is even an increased comfort with my body. However, perhaps the biggest eye-opener for me during the workshop was facing my beliefs about love. I realized I was still holding some negative attitudes about how love manifests. Today I affirm that love is God's indelible creation, love is who I am and all of us are. –Carol, TX

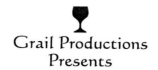

Grail Productions
Presents

— WORKSHOP FEEDBACK —

There are a number of changes that have occurred for me and through me during and since the workshop. The love I feel is exhilarating. I now see my body as beautiful. I stopped judging my imperfections and see myself for the beautiful child of God I am. Through the many exercises during the workshop, I was able to connect with my body in a way I had never done before. Now I am constantly feeling my whole body, and it's great–there is no numbness, just pure loving energy! I also released many of my issues of shame–shame of my body and of who I am. I also learned that each loving moment is perfect in itself and that intimacy does not have to progress to sex. For me, this is liberating and beautiful. –Joelle, FL

Grail Productions
Presents

ORDER FORM

To order *Sacred Sexuality, A Manual for Living Bliss* or *The Seven Initiations of the Spiritual Path* or to request more information on either of these publications, please complete and send or fax in the order form below.

You can also visit our website (www.grailproductions.com) for a complete list of books and tapes (audio and video).

Name_____

Address_____

City, State, Zip_____

Phone_____

Fax_____

Email_____

Please include any special instructions when ordering.
Please make checks payable to: Grail Productions

_____

_____

_____

Sacred Sexuality, A Manual for Living Bliss
_____ copies at $25.00 each =   _____

The Seven Initiations of the Spiritual Path
_____ copies at $15.00 each =   _____

Add $2.00 for S&H per book   _____

Total   _____

Grail Productions, PO Box 2783, Bellingham, WA 98227
For information: (360) 671-8349 or **grailpro@aol.com**.
Visit us at **www.grailproductions.com**

CPSIA information can be obtained
at www.ICGtesting.com
Printed in the USA
FFOW03n0147311215
19767FF